Everything must change

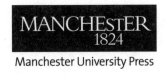

MANCHESTER
1824

Manchester University Press

Everything must change

Philosophical lessons from lockdown

Vittorio Bufacchi

Manchester University Press

The right of Vittorio Bufacchi to be identified as the author of this
work has been asserted by them in accordance with the Copyright,
Designs and Patents Act 1988.

Published by Manchester University Press
Altrincham Street, Manchester M1 7JA
www.manchesteruniversitypress.co.uk

British Library Cataloguing-in-Publication Data
A catalogue record for this book is available from the British Library

ISBN 978 1 5261 5877 2 hardback

First published 2021

The publisher has no responsibility for the persistence or accuracy of
URLs for any external or third-party internet websites referred to in
this book, and does not guarantee that any content on such websites is,
or will remain, accurate or appropriate.

Typeset by
Servis Filmsetting Ltd, Stockport, Cheshire
Printed in Great Britain by
Bell and Bain Ltd, Glasgow

For
Natalie and Jacobo

Contents

Preface

'If you have a garden and a library, you have everything you need.' So said the Roman philosopher Marcus Tullius Cicero (106–43 BCE), and he was right. During the weeks of lockdown in March and April 2020, forced upon us by the COVID-19 pandemic, what made the experience tolerable for me was the fact that at home I had the luxury of a library and a garden. In this I know I'm very lucky.

This book was written in the months between March and November 2020, as the pandemic advanced and a strange new world unfolded. It stems from my desire to make sense of extraordinary events with the help of the only tool at my disposal: philosophical analysis. Throughout this period, I was always fully aware of the fortunate position I found myself in, and how luck, or to be precise the lack of it, is perhaps the greatest contributor to social injustice. I had my books, a garden, my health, and a family around me. I also had financial security due to my ability to work from home.

The impact of COVID-19 is not the same for everyone. This crisis magnifies every existing inequality, exposing the dynamics of social injustice in every community and society. People with small children, or whose children have special needs, are expected to 'work from home' by management structures oblivious to the reality of diverse social contexts. People who live in fear of violence are expected to share the same confined space with their abusers. People with no income are overlooked. The aim of this book is to record, expose, and analyse some of these realities of the pandemic.

Apart from giving me time and space to write this book, the lockdown was good to me in another way. It gave me the most unexpected gift: time to connect with and get to know my teenage children. This book is dedicated to them, Natalie and Jacobo. They belong to 'the next generation', those who will inherit from us a world bursting with injustice, inequality, and for too many people, hopelessness. I can only hope that they will do a better job of it than my generation.

Some material for this book appeared, in a very different and more impulsive form, in articles I wrote for a number of outlets including *RTÉ Brainstorm*, *The Conversation UK*, *Irish Examiner*, *Global-e*, and the *New Statesman*. I also used snippets of arguments I published in the following two articles: 'Justice as non-maleficence', *Theoria*, 67.162 (2020), and 'Truth, lies and tweets: a consensus theory of post-truth', *Philosophy & Social Criticism* (first published online 14 January 2020). I thank the publishers for permission to use the material here.

Preface

I was lucky to share the experience of the lockdown with my wife and companion of the last twenty years, Jools Gilson. She was with me every step of the way, every minute of the day, and I cherished every moment. We played cards with the children, we turned our lawn into raised beds for our vegetables, and we learned from each other how to navigate uncharted waters. She was, and always will be, the only person I wish to spend an extended period of isolation with.

Emma Brennan at Manchester University Press deserves special praise. She is the kind of editor any author would wish for. Always supportive and impeccably efficient, this book benefited immensely from her nurturing input at all stages of the publication process. I'm also very grateful to an anonymous reviewer who gave me extremely detailed feedback on the whole manuscript. Thank you, whoever you are.

Towards the end of this project two of my best students, Ellen Byrne and Órla McCarthy, helped me with some additional research, sharp scrutiny of my argument, and much-needed editorial advice. They did sterling work, and I'm very grateful to them.

Finally, Helen Beebee was exceptionally kind in offering to read the entire manuscript. Words cannot capture my indebtedness to her, but sadly it will be some time before I can express my gratitude in the proper way: with a pint of Murphy's in an Irish pub with Six Nations rugby on the television in the background. Her sharp comments and suggestions were invaluable, and her encouragement has always been immeasurable. To be able to call Helen a friend reminds me of another quote from Cicero: 'Without true friend-ship, life is nothing.'

St Luke's, Cork
November 2020

Coronavirus and philosophy

> There have been as many plagues as wars in history;
> yet always plagues and wars take people equally by
> surprise.
>
> Albert Camus, The Plague

The Roman philosopher Marcus Tullius Cicero famously said that 'to study philosophy is nothing but to prepare one's self to die'.[1] Cicero wrote this in 45 BCE in a text of philosophical ruminations known as *Tusculan Disputations*. In the first book of this philosophical treatise Cicero challenges the widely held belief that death is an evil, and thus to be feared.

As I write this introduction, death is inescapably on my mind, and probably on the mind of many readers. The reason, needless to say, is COVID-19, caused by the SARS-CoV-2 virus or more colloquially coronavirus; whatever its name, this highly infectious disease caused by a severe acute respiratory syndrome is the most devastating and lethal pandemic in living memory. At present, 47 million cases of the virus have been reported, causing the deaths of more than 1.2 million people worldwide.[2] By the time you read these pages these numbers will be even more frightening, and the pain and fear left in the virus's wake unspeakable. Eight times more people have died in New York City from COVID-19 than from the terrorist attack on 9/11. More people have died in the UK from COVID-19 than were killed in the Blitz during the Second World War. COVID-19 has made the fear of death tangible to everyone, everywhere in the world.

Cicero had a very specific reason for wanting to apply his considerable philosophical skills to the subject of death. A few months before he wrote *Tusculan Disputations* his beloved daughter Tullia died, at the age of 34, during childbirth. Cicero never recovered from the grief, and the pain he endured shattered his personal life. Soon after the death of Tullia he divorced his second wife Publilia, whom he had married only the previous year, allegedly because she couldn't comprehend the agony he was suffering. Cicero was himself assassinated two years later.[3]

To ease the pain Cicero turned to philosophy. In the first book of *Tusculan Disputations* he uses logical reasoning to convince the reader that death is not to be feared: if death brings nothingness, there is literally 'nothing' to fear, and if death takes us to an eternal afterlife, then far from fearing death, we should welcome it. For Cicero what is much more difficult to accept, and to come to terms with, is not our own death but the loss of those we love. Thus, the second and third books of *Tusculan Disputations* are respectively on the subject of bearing pain and grief. Ultimately,

Tusculan Disputations is Cicero's love letter to his departed daughter.

Similarly, the unfolding global tragedy of COVID-19 is something we cannot escape. The numbers of the deceased are so great as to become mere statistics, and it is all too easy to forget that behind each and every death there are many who despair, like Cicero, for the loss of a friend, a father or a mother, a wife or a husband, or indeed a son or a daughter. This is why we need philosophy. Like Cicero more than 2,000 years ago, we look to philosophy to conquer the fear of death. And as we make our way through a new reality that many of us have never experienced, we turn to philosophy to help us make (some) sense of the absurdity that is around us.

Cicero was an immense influence on many philosophers over many centuries, especially during the period of humanism, or to be precise Renaissance humanism, an intellectual movement in Europe of the later Middle Ages and the Early Modern period. One of the most significant thinkers in the humanist tradition was the French philosopher Michel de Montaigne (1533–92), the author of a famous essay entitled 'That to Study Philosophy is to Learn to Die'.[4] The influence of Cicero on Montaigne is undeniable. But Montaigne takes his analysis of death in a totally different direction to Cicero. According to Montaigne, it is not just the case that we need to understand death before we can hope to make sense of life, but that comprehending death is the key to the very *art of living*. Montaigne

3

captures this idea in typically exuberant style: 'He who has learned how to die has unlearned how to be a slave.'[5]

Montaigne is not making a banal assertion that portrays the Grim Reaper as our master and we, mere mortals, as its slaves. Instead, what Montaigne is telling us is that what keeps us enslaved is the fear of death, the terror of our annihilation. Liberty is the opposite of domination, and as long as we live our lives under the dominion of the anxiety of death, we are never truly free. It is only when we learn to welcome death's approach that we become free. But to achieve this freedom will take time, and effort, and a great deal of philosophy.

In the most abrupt and unexpected way, coronavirus has forced us to reflect on this most basic aspect of the human condition: our mortality. The fear of catching the virus, and of the unknown repercussions this may have on our lives, has made us reflect on our mortality in a way that no one had anticipated or expected.

For many months now, starting in February 2020, death and COVID-19 have been ever-present on every television channel and radio station when the news comes on. Death, or the fear of death, is still on the front pages of all the newspapers. In learning to live with coronavirus we are trapped in a catch-22: we want to escape this state of anxiety, but in staying responsibly informed we cannot get away from it. Perhaps Montaigne had the right solution: we cannot run away from death, we cannot pretend that death doesn't concern us, therefore we have no choice but to face death head-on:

> We must learn to stand firm and to fight it. To begin depriving death of its greatest advantage over us, let us adopt a way clean contrary to that common one; let us deprive death of its strangeness; let us frequent it, let us get used to it; let us have nothing more often in mind than death. At every instant let us evoke it in our imagination under all its aspects. Whenever a horse stumbles, a tile falls or a pin pricks however lightly, let us at once chew over this thought: 'Supposing that was death itself?' With that, let us brace ourselves and make an effort. In the midst of joy and feasting let our refrain be one which recalls our human condition.[6]

Montaigne was right: facing our mortality is the only way to properly learn the 'art of living'. This is something we can take from the present crisis. Coronavirus has given us an opportunity that may not come again. Trapped in the relentless hectic rhythm of modern life, always multi-tasking, forever chasing the evanescent gold standard of productivity, we have forgotten about the art of living.

And so, while death will be a recurring theme, this book is not about death but about the art of living.[7] More specifically, it is about the *politics* and the *ethics* of the art of living. The focus of this book will be on what we can learn from the experience of living with COVID-19, as individuals but also collectively as a society. More specifically, this book starts from the premise that this deadly crisis could potentially change our lives for the better, ushering in a more just society.

I will be looking at eight coronavirus-related themes through philosophical lenses, one in each of the chapters that follow. Chapter 2 will ask the question whether coronavirus is a misfortune or an injustice. It is tempting, and oddly reassuring, to think of this virus-induced crisis as a global misfortune, something that could not have been predicted, or anticipated, and that no one can be blamed for. Like an earthquake or a hurricane, this virus is merely an act of nature, and the only thing we can do is defend ourselves from the whims of misfortune as best we can. But there is another way to look at this crisis: it has fully exposed the chronic social injustice that pervades our modern society. The response to this crisis is also imbued with serious issues of global social injustice.

Chapter 3 will focus on the largest cohort of victims of coronavirus: people living in old age. This crisis has forced us to rethink the way society sees people over the age of 65, and the often inadequate and disrespectful way in which our productivity-obsessed modern world shows contempt for its more senior members, to a great extent because of their perceived waning autonomy.

Chapter 4 will attempt to answer the question whether life under coronavirus is comparable to life in the so-called 'state of nature'. The state of nature is a term of art for political philosophers, and the reference here is specifically to the work of Thomas Hobbes, an English philosopher who wrote his masterpiece *Leviathan* towards the end of the Civil War in 1651.

For Hobbes, the state of nature is a place of abysmal anarchy, where we live in incessant fear of oblivion, and where life is 'solitary, poor, nasty, brutish, and short'. We are not in a state of nature, not yet anyway, but there are elements of Hobbes's state of nature that resemble certain aspects of our lives under enforced lockdown, marked by uncertainty as they are. The chapter will also evaluate ways to leave, or avoid, a full-scale state of nature.

Chapter 5 will explore the impact of coronavirus on the global phenomenon of populism, which had become the dominant ideology up to the outbreak of the pandemic. The question we need to ask ourselves is whether populism will come out of this crisis weaker or stronger than it was before. While the jury is still out on this question, and only time will tell, the chapter suggests that populism could be one of the major victims of this pandemic.

Populism, especially of its right-wing variety, is never far from propelling fake news, and its political leaders tend to be enthusiastic champions of post-truth. One of the features of the present crisis has been the extent to which all sorts of half-truths and outright lies have been allowed to spread. Chapter 6 will explore the relationship between post-truth and coronavirus, and it will suggest things that we can learn from this crisis in the fight against post-truth.

Chapter 7 will focus on the role of arguably the most important players in the response to the coronavirus pandemic: the experts. The World Health Organization

(WHO) has been at the forefront of the fight against the virus, and every country has its own team of scientific experts: epidemiologists, virologists, microbiologists, and the mathematicians with their sophisticated models. The problem is that experts don't always agree with each other, there isn't always one, unanimous, uncontested scientific truth. This raises a set of important questions. Who do we trust? And what do we base our trust on?

Chapter 8 will look at one of the most disturbing aspects of the lockdown experience: worldwide there has been a 25 per cent increase in recorded incidents of domestic violence. The issue of domestic violence will be addressed via an analysis of Sally Rooney's award-winning novel *Normal People*, which was turned into a successful television adaptation by the BBC and aired during lockdown in April 2020 in Ireland and the UK.

Finally, the concluding chapter will argue that there is one principal lesson to be learned from this pandemic: that politics is not only important, but essential, and often the main difference between life and death. In politics, mixing incompetence with hubris can be lethal, not for the politicians but for the general public. More specifically, this pandemic has reminded us of three key political certainties: the necessity of the state to coordinate social efforts; the requirement to raise taxes to facilitate the essential work that only the state can carry out; and the imperative to introduce new radical social and economic reforms, including a universal basic income.

2

COVID-19:
injustice or misfortune?

Yes, there was an element of abstraction and unreality in misfortune. But when an abstraction starts to kill you, you have to get to work on it.

Albert Camus, *The Plague*

There are two ways to think of a human tragedy: as a (social) injustice or as a misfortune. A misfortune is usually associated with inescapable external forces of nature, and as such the desolation it leaves in its wake is blameless. The devastating impact of a hurricane, or the trauma of a brain tumour, are dreadful, awful realities, but as acts of nature they can be deemed mere misfortunes. An injustice, on the other hand, is caused by fellow humans, not nature. An injustice, unlike a misfortune, is intentional, controllable, and therefore not blameless. Poverty is an injustice, not a misfortune. The impact of COVID-19 has a lot more to do with injustice than misfortune.

At an intuitive level this distinction between an injustice and a misfortune makes sense, and yet actually distinguishing between the two can be profoundly problematic.[1] In her still relevant book *The Faces of Injustice*, first published thirty years ago, Judith Shklar reminds us that what is a misfortune to one is an injustice to another, and the perception of what is an injustice as opposed to a misfortune will often differ if it is described by the victim or the bystander.[2]

Perceptions of injustice are a powerful tool in our effort to make sense of the world we live in. To those not directly affected, the destruction of a school by an earthquake might seem like a quintessential case of misfortune; but to the families of the victims who were told the school was built to withstand an earthquake, this is a case of injustice. Flooding in Bangladesh or the rising sea level in the Maldives might be conveniently dismissed as misfortunes; alternatively, the unequal impact of climate change suggests that in fact we are looking at cases of environmental global injustice.

But things are not as simple as they might seem. Shklar goes on to warn us that perceptions of injustice must be taken with a pinch of salt, and she is right about this. We must take the victims' views seriously; however, this does not mean that victims are always right when they perceive injustice. When things go wrong, and the unspeakable occurs, often our only way to cope is to find someone to blame – or, as Shklar says, we blame anyone who seems more fortunate than ourselves.[3]

What is social injustice?

Of course, this doesn't mean that perceptions of injustice are always wrong, or that it is never a case of injustice but only of misfortune. But it does mean that we desperately need a theory of social injustice to test the validity of our intuitions. And this is where philosophy has an important role to play. Since the time of Plato political philosophers have asked the question 'What is justice?' This is perhaps the dominant question driving the entire discipline of political philosophy. John Rawls, arguably the greatest and most influential political philosopher since John Stuart Mill in the nineteenth century, is absolutely right when he states that social justice is the first virtue of social institutions, as truth is of systems of thought.[4] But one unintended consequence of asking 'What is justice?' has been that 'social injustice' has continually lived in the shadow of its more glamorous twin, 'social justice'. In recent years the quest for the philosophical coordinates of a just society has resulted in the advent of one of the most productive and lucrative industries in the academic profession, while the idea of social injustice has been almost universally neglected, being dismissed as conceptually uninteresting. After all, isn't social injustice simply the lack, absence, or negation of social justice? Doesn't social justice tell us everything we need to know about social injustice, the latter being merely the negative side of the former?

The short answer is 'No'. There are two ways to approach the concept of social injustice. The dominant approach suggests that social injustice is simply the opposite of social justice. According to this view social justice and social injustice are mutually defined opposites, with social justice performing the dominant role, while the concept of social injustice is relegated to that of a negative by-product. The assumption is that if we know what constitutes justice, then we automatically know everything we need to know about social injustice, since social injustice is lurking wherever something or someone impedes the realization of our ideal.

But there is another way to think about social injustice. We must resist the arbitrary dictates of etymology, theorizing injustice as a sheer negation of something else.[5] We ought to think of social injustice independently of our conception of social justice. Instead of assuming that social justice comes first while social injustice is derivative of justice, we should turn things on their head: social justice is the absence of social injustice, not the other way around.[6] As I argued in my book *Social Injustice*,[7] the trick is to think of justice and injustice in terms of the relationship between 'solution' and 'problem': social injustice is the problem, and social justice the solution. It is nonsensical to discuss solutions before we know the nature of the problem; similarly we cannot articulate the demands of social justice unless we have a grasp of the nature of social injustice. For these reasons, it is imperative not only to take social injustice seriously, but conceptually to prioritize social injustice over social justice, relegating theories of social justice to a by-product of our theories about injustice rather than vice versa, as widely assumed.

Which brings us back to the question: is coronavirus a misfortune or an injustice? In terms of the timing and the molecular structure of this particular infectious virus there are elements of misfortune, but the unequal impact of COVID-19 is certainly an injustice, since as we will see some groups have been affected much worse than others, and arbitrarily so. Certain underlying aspects of our unjust society have been magnified and fully exposed by COVID-19, starting from the gross inequalities that are a constant feature of every facet of the social order.

However, in order to appreciate why COVID-19 has a lot more to do with social injustice than misfortune, we need to say a little more about social injustice. Ideally we would need a full theory of social injustice, but short of that, an appreciation of the key dimensions of social injustice will suffice. Only then will we be able to assess whether our perceptions of injustice are accurate or misguided.

There are two ways of thinking about social injustice: as an act of domination, with externally imposed restrictions on our freedom, in particular our freedom to act on our choices and desires. Alternatively, social injustice can take the form of oppression, which curtails our self-expression; in other words it restrains our ambitions, dreams, and expectations like an invisible straitjacket. Domination tends to be the prevalent way of thinking about social injustice, but this conception is also very narrow, and potentially misleading; it could even justify the actions of armed militia groups protesting against COVID-19 lockdowns in places such as Michigan, who choose to see the temporary state of emergency as an affront to basic freedoms and thus as an act of tyranny by the central authority.

In her book *Justice and the Politics of Difference*, Iris M. Young explains how oppression is much more subtle, and as such can take many forms.[8] Oppression refers to structural phenomena that immobilize or diminish a group. Her emphasis on the structural or institutional nature of social injustice is critically important, and accurate. It reminds us that social injustice cannot be reduced to the intentional act of an individual aimed at harming another person; instead it is in-built in the socio-economic system itself. So although some people are chronically disadvantaged and overpowered, there isn't always a specific person or group that can be blamed for this state of affairs. Racism is an example of oppression as structural injustice, as the Black Lives Matter movement is assiduously trying to point out: police brutality is not a single incident of domination, but the expression of institutionalized oppression against black people and other minorities.[9]

Oppression manifests itself in many different ways, including exploitation, marginalization, powerlessness, cultural imperialism, and violence. These are what Young refers to as the five categories of oppression, even though as she herself admits, these five categories of oppression do not constitute a full theory of social injustice.

A full account of the nature of social injustice cannot be separated from the question of motivation; in other words, we cannot separate the question 'What is injustice?' from the question 'Why be unjust?'[10] There is a simple answer to the latter question: for the sake of power. The more complex answer reminds us that power is a relative concept to be understood within a social context. Being in power means having power *over others*. The best way to acquire power is to take power away from others, and the best way to maintain power is to acquire more control of resources than others, and in the process to disempower others.

I suggest that we theorize social injustice in terms of a three-dimensional framework, according to which an injustice is constituted by three separate but interacting facets: maldistribution, exclusion, and disempowerment.[11] All three dimensions are at work whenever there is an injustice, even though, depending on the specific instance of injustice under consideration, one of the three dimensions may turn out to be more dominant than the other two.

Maldistribution is the improper or injurious distribution of resources across society. An injustice occurs when material and social resources are distributed according to criteria that not everyone (especially those who stand to receive less than others) could reasonably accept.

Exclusion refers to actions or policies undertaken to exclude on arbitrary grounds certain members of society from being legitimate recipients of the distribution of benefits and burdens that arises from social cooperation.

Disempowerment occurs when the social or economic vulnerabilities of a group in society are exposed and exploited. Disempowerment is not to be confused with powerlessness: while powerlessness defines the lack of power of one group in relation to another group, disempowerment is the process whereby a group gradually loses its influence, and impact, in a decision process that affects it directly. Victims of social injustice are disempowered by the experience of injustice, in the sense that their powers are diminished, and therefore they become increasingly vulnerable to suffering further injustice in the future. In Ireland the victims of industrial schools and workhouses such as the Magdalene Laundries were not only exploited and abused, both physically and psychologically, but they were put in a position where it was impossible for them to demand justice, even many decades after the events.[12]

What makes social injustice in modern society particularly insidious is the fact that injustice is no longer exercised via brute force, as in the past. We are past the age of might-makes-right. Instead, social injustice today works in elusive, obscure ways. Those who suffer from poverty, those who are unemployed, or those who have no choice but to take on many different part-time jobs just to keep their heads above water, are now being blamed for their predicament. The fact that poverty tends to have a specific social profile, based on race or gender or ethnicity or religion for example, is simply dismissed as irrelevant. The chronic and institutionalized forms of maldistribution, exclusion, and disempowerment are rarely considered as part of the explanation of why some people are disadvantaged. The myth of meritocracy not only succeeds in justifying the achievements of those at the top, but it also puts the blame for some people's lack of success on to their own alleged inadequacies. We have built our society around the implausible, unfathomable lie that poverty is the just reward for being lazy, stupid, unmotivated, or merely lacking ambition.[13]

The global injustice of COVID-19

There are two ways to measure the injustice of COVID-19: globally and domestically. As the virus progressed from an epidemic to a pandemic, those of us living in affluent societies were told that one of the most effective lines of defence at our disposal was self-isolation, and washing our hands, repeatedly, with soap. This seems easy, until you realize that globally things are different. According to a report from the World Health Organization from June 2019, some 3 billion people around the world lack basic handwashing facilities.[14]

In developing countries, three-quarters of the population live in 'slums', where a slum is defined by overcrowding, poor or informal housing, inadequate access to safe water and sanitation, and insecurity of tenure. As Mike Davis tells us in his detailed account of slums, 'there were at least 921 million slum-dwellers in 2001: nearly equal to the population of the world when the young Engels first ventured onto the mean streets of Manchester'.[15]

The reference here is to Friedrich Engels, close friend of Karl Marx, but more importantly the author of *The Condition of the Working Class in England*, first published in 1845. Engels gives a gruesome and disturbing account of how hundreds of thousands of people in the north of England lived so that a few wealthy capitalists could reap the benefits of their labour. Engels explains how the dwellings of working people were in streets generally unpaved, rough, dirty, filled with vegetable and animal refuse, without sewers or gutters, but supplied with foul, stagnant pools instead. Moreover, there was almost no ventilation. Engels failed to see how any human being could possibly wish to live in these houses, overcrowded and filthy within and without. In these houses lived children who were deprived of their childhood because they had to work, some from the age of 7, up to 60 hours a week. As Engels explained: 'Women made unfit for child-bearing, children deformed, men enfeebled, limbs crushed, whole generations wrecked, afflicted with disease and infirmity, purely to fill the purses of the bourgeoisie.'[16]

We cannot read about Engels's Manchester today without a feeling of shame and rage prompted by a profound sense of injustice. These are the same emotions we feel when we read the novels of Elizabeth Gaskell, also set in Manchester in the 1840s, especially *Mary Barton*, *Ruth*, and *North and South*. But the truth is that very little has changed since then, except that the most extreme misery and exploitation are not on our doorsteps any more. Modern capitalism still needs the cheap labour of millions of people, but it has learned to outsource it to places where the wealthy cannot see this misery.

What hope have millions of people in the poorest countries in the world of escaping the worst effects of this virus, given their living conditions? Like the nineteenth-century proletarian from Engels's time, 'who has nothing but his two hands, who consumes today what he earned yesterday, who is subject to every possible chance, and has not the slightest guarantee for being able to earn the barest necessities of life, whom every crisis, every whim of his employer may deprive of bread',[17] millions of people today are left with nothing and nowhere to hide. Engels told us that the proletarian 'is placed in the most revolting, inhuman position conceivable for a human being'.[18] Globally speaking, we have not made any progress since the 1840s.

Home to just 8 per cent of the global population, in June 2020 Latin America was suffering half the world's new coronavirus deaths. The poverty and inequality in Latin America, which forces most of its population to make a living from the informal economy, is a primary reason for this recent development.

Consider Brazil. 13.6 million people live in favelas or shanty-towns in Brazil, roughly 6 per cent of the population, in overcrowded accommodation often lacking basic sanitation. People living here cannot isolate, they cannot wash their hands, and if they don't work they don't eat. Gilson Rodrigues, community leader in Paraisópolis, the largest favela in São Paulo, expected the worst: 'It is here that we will have more cases [of COVID-19], in the favelas. How can an old person self-isolate in a house with ten people and two rooms? This isolation is a joke; it is for the rich. The poor cannot do it. We are going to lose a lot of people in the favelas, sadly.'[19] Brazil had 5 million cases of COVID-19 and 150,000 deaths by October 2020, the second highest in the world (after the USA).

The devastating impact of COVID-19 on Kenya, especially for women, is also under-reported. When COVID-19 lockdown hit Kenya in March 2020, the resurgence of a different – this time man-made – epidemic followed in its wake. As schools closed across the country, reports surged of young girls being forced to undergo marriage, female genital mutilation (FGM), and early pregnancy. Lockdown poverty has taken a severe toll on many already-struggling communities, where some underage girls have been forced into transactional sex just to buy food. Desperate families have resorted to marrying off their young daughters for the sake of valuable dowries, with some of these girls undergoing FGM as part of traditional pre-marriage customs. In addition, with the closure of the safe haven of schools, reports of sexual violence – including child rape – have increased exponentially. One Kenyan county has reported more than 4,000 cases of early pregnancy since March. Although child marriage has been prohibited in Kenya since its ratification of the UN Convention on the Rights of the Child in 1990, many children's rights groups fear that progress made in this regard is being rapidly eroded; one national helpline has reported a more than tenfold increase in calls since lockdown began, increasing from 86 in February to over 1,100 in June.[20]

In the last analysis, the poor are more exposed and susceptible to disease, less capable of accessing healthcare when they catch the virus, and thus more likely to pass it on. As Octávio Luiz Motta Ferraz points out, the poor bear a disproportionate burden of morbidity and mortality, explained by three main disadvantages caused by poverty. First, differential exposure: unfavourable living and working conditions, and lack of education. Second, differential susceptibility: worse underlying health conditions associated with poverty, such as malnutrition, psychological stress, high blood pressure, diabetes, and heart disease. And third, differential access to healthcare.

The virus will have a devastating effect on all poorer nations, not just Brazil, and the reason for this is the precarious conditions of poverty that millions of people find themselves in. David Malpass, the head of the World Bank, has warned that the COVID-19 crisis could push another 60 million people into poverty worldwide, while according to Oxfam 121 million more people face being pushed to the brink of starvation because of the COVID-19 pandemic.[21]

Injustice in the West

In wealthier nations things are better, but only marginally. Gender, class, race, and disability are still determining factors in the identity of those worst affected by COVID-19. From domestic violence to bearing the brunt of lay-offs, women have been disproportionately affected by the COVID-19 pandemic. And as if this wasn't bad enough, their voices and expertise are being ignored. Research conducted by the Global Institute for Women's Leadership at King's College London shows that for every mention of a prominent woman expert in COVID-19 coverage, there are nineteen mentions of a man.[22] Miranda Fricker calls this prevalent phenomenon 'epistemic injustice'; this is a special kind of injustice that arises when someone wrongly treats someone else as a poor source of information, usually because of prejudice towards a particular group.[23]

Pandemics strike hardest where there is inequality and poverty, and predictably COVID-19 has had a different impact depending on the status and social class of citizens. There is a clear class and race divide in the COVID-19 death rate, with those in low-paid, working-class jobs clearly worse affected than those in middle- and upper-class jobs, where people had the luxury to self-isolate and work from home.[24] And of course low-paid, working-class jobs are not equally distributed across ethnic and racial groups. Minority ethnic groups account for 34 per cent of critically ill COVID-19 patients in the UK despite constituting 14 per cent of the population. One possible explanation for this is that patients of black, Asian, and minority ethnicity live in overcrowded and poor standard homes in geographical areas where air pollution is highest.[25] In the UK, the Office for National Statistics has estimated that disabled women are 2.4 times more likely to die from COVID-19 than non-disabled women, and disabled men 1.9 times more likely to die than non-disabled men.[26]

Nurses, historically among the worst-paid members of the health system, have been expected to go out to work in hospitals and care homes even without adequate protection, as were cleaners and other manual labourers. In the United States, black Americans are dying of COVID-19 at three times the rate of white people.[27] In Poland coal mines have been badly hit by coronavirus, since social distancing is impossible in the mines. Of the country's more than 36,000 reported infections, about 6,500 are miners, meaning that miners constitute nearly one-fifth of all confirmed cases. Across Europe food delivery riders are another category of workers who were expected to work during the crisis, since food delivery was considered an essential activity; however, they were not given face masks, they do not have the luxury of any labour rights, and they are among the lowest-paid workers in our economy.[28]

Because of the precarious nature of work in advanced capitalist societies, scores of people had no choice but to go to work, notwithstanding the high risk to their health. For example, bus drivers suffered a staggeringly high rate of infection. Many other workers lost their jobs overnight, and with it their entire well-being and that of their families. In Ireland, the meat industry is renowned for the stringent health and safety measures surrounding its products, but the people who process those products are not afforded the same consideration. After scores of clusters of infections across Ireland and Europe, the real dangers of the meat industry are being exposed: low wages, extreme working hours, subcontracting, lack of unionization and lack of sick pay. The decision to report symptoms is inevitably impacted when 80–90 per cent of workers do not have sick pay to fall back on, and 41 per cent of the migrant workers in the industry are non-EU citizens whose residency depends on employment. In Denmark, only a handful of COVID-19 cases have been reported in the meat industry. The meat industry sector in Denmark is characterized by health and safety precautions, strong union membership and no subcontracting. Austria and Sweden have employed similar measures to Denmark and have witnessed similar results.

In Europe and the United States, we had the good fortune of prior warning, a luxury that the inhabitants of the Hubei region in China did not have. And yet adequate measures were not implemented, with deadly delays and hesitations. In the UK mistakes were made on almost a daily basis. The government's policy for the procurement of ventilators badly backfired, with the minimum specification for the UK's homegrown hospital ventilator programme deemed unsuitable for treating coronavirus patients.[29] A shipment from Turkey of 400,000 units of personal protective equipment for health workers was found not to conform to UK standards, and returned.[30] And then there was the very high rate of contagions and deaths in care homes for older citizens; the impact of COVID-19 on old age and care homes will be discussed in greater detail in Chapter 3.

The slowness of many Western countries to prepare and respond to this crisis, chiefly the UK and the US, reveals something about social injustice in these countries. We said before that to get a grasp of social injustice we must not only answer the question 'What is injustice?', but also the question 'Why be unjust?' The botched response to this crisis in the UK and the US says a great deal about the motivations of injustice of the political class in these two countries.[31]

The prospect of shutting down the economy, even only temporarily, to save lives was always going to be the last resort for Boris Johnson and Donald Trump. Their motivation for maintaining the status quo was simple: to keep things as they are, not rock the boat, and not endanger their own personal interests. After all, they are global leaders in a world where, according to an Oxfam report from 2018, 82 per cent of the wealth generated that year went to the richest 1 per cent of the global population, while the 3.7 billion people who make up the poorer half of the world saw no increase in their wealth.[32] In the US the top 1 per cent are close to surpassing the wealth of the entire middle class, while the poorest have 35 per cent of the liabilities but just 6 per cent of the assets.[33] In the UK, the share of income enjoyed by the top 1 per cent has generally been rising, peaking to 13 per cent in 2015.[34] And of course, it is this top 1 per cent who are the main financial donors to the Republican Party and the Conservative Party respectively. In the UK, almost one-third of the UK's richest people have donated almost £52m to the Conservative Party, while almost £100bn has been handed back in tax breaks to the super-rich and big corporations.[35]

The only way to cope with COVID-19 was to make some radical decisions. Yes, the economy was going to suffer, and yes, it was going to be very expensive to provide emergency payments to people who were unable to work while the country was in lockdown. Who was going to pay for this? The obvious answer should be the top 1 per cent, or perhaps the top 30 per cent. To some of our political leaders this was unacceptable, inconceivable, which is why in the UK Boris Johnson was flirting with 'herd immunity' as a strategy, and why Donald Trump dismissed the pandemic as a hoax. Their motivation was clear: to maintain the status quo and accordingly their own interests, at all costs, even that of many human lives. The fact that the status quo is structurally unjust, as evidenced by the growing chasm between the top 1 per cent and the rest of society, was not a concern.

Conclusion

COVID-19 has fully exposed the true character of our society: its remorseless injustice. Compared to 2019, in the first six months of 2020 the UK registered the highest percentage increase of deaths in Europe. These deaths were not caused by misfortune, but by injustice.[36]

At the start of this crisis, one might have been tempted to be fatalistic; indeed in recent months there has been a revival of interest in the philosophy of Stoicism, which teaches us to accept all things that are beyond the power of our will. The first-century Roman philosopher Seneca made a clear distinction between experiencing a setback and suffering from it: following his teachings, we must learn to cease worrying about COVID-19, or the risk of death, and experience the unfolding events with serenity.[37]

The truth about COVID-19 is much more complex, and much less reassuring. No one is responsible for the fact that viruses exist, nor for the fact that some viruses are more harmful than others; but collectively we are responsible for the fact that pandemic preparedness plans were grossly insufficient, and the response to the crisis almost totally inadequate. Not to mention the fact that in the UK, Ireland, and many other countries, many years of privatization and austerity have left society ill-prepared to deal with a major crisis. This is where injustice creeps in.

This is not the time to dabble with Stoicism, but to embrace Critical Theory: what we need is social inquiry aimed at human emancipation, especially given the present context of domination and oppression. The structural injustice of modern society, where a tiny minority benefits disproportionately at the expense of the rest of humanity, and where the political class puts the interests of the top 1 per cent of wealthiest people before the other 99 per cent of the population, has been magnified for all to see. All the inequalities, biases, prejudices, and wrongs of modern society have been irrevocably exposed by COVID-19.

3

Old age in the time of coronavirus

… well-meaning speakers tried to voice their fellow-feeling, and indeed did so, but at the same time proved the utter incapacity of every man truly to share in suffering which he cannot see.

Albert Camus, *The Plague*

We live in an ageing society. In 2017 the United Nations noted the following trends in global population ageing:

- The global population aged 60 years or over numbered 962 million in 2017, more than twice as large as in 1980, when there were 382 million older persons worldwide.
- The number of older persons is expected to double again by 2050, when it is projected to reach nearly 2.1 billion.
- Globally, the number of persons aged 80 years or over is projected to increase more than threefold between 2017 and 2050, rising from 137 million to 425 million.[1]

Whoever compiled these statistics had not anticipated a respiratory pandemic that disproportionately affects the elderly: the average age of death from COVID-19 is over 80, and 80 per cent of the infected Chinese who died were aged 60 and older. Estimates of the worst-case scenario vary, but more than two million people worldwide will die from COVID-19 unless a vaccine is developed. The majority of them will be over 60.

Most health systems around the world could not cope with the surge of COVID-19 related cases. In 2018 in Ireland there were only 6 critical care beds (including beds in private hospitals) per 100,000 population compared with the European average of 11.5 per 100,000. Managing the COVID-19 crisis required both medical and ethical expertise. The Italian College of Anaesthesia, Analgesia, Resuscitation and Intensive Care (SIAARTI) published guidelines for the criteria that doctors and nurses should follow when making decisions about life and death. Perhaps not surprisingly, the utilitarian principle of maximizing benefit for the largest number of people was invoked. Also not surprisingly, but more alarmingly, medical staff were told to consider the age of the patients before allocating ventilators: 'It may become necessary to establish an age limit for access to intensive care.'[2] Similar guidelines were being considered in the US.[3]

While these criteria may be shocking, they are not immoral. In a context of scarcity of resources some objective (or at least not subjective) criteria are necessary when prioritizing patients. The utilitarian calculations adopted by SIAARTI were not unprecedented. Similar criteria apply in the context of organ donation, where patients are ranked on waiting lists using a calculation of the chances of the transplant's success and the patient's survival.[4]

But in the UK, policy guidelines took a more sinister turn. The idea that old people could be sacrificed for the sake of the common good appeared to be the guiding principle before the policy of herd immunity was aborted. At a private event at the end of February, Boris Johnson's chief adviser Dominic Cummings allegedly said that the government's strategy at the time could be summarized in the following terms: 'herd immunity, protect the economy, and if that means some pensioners die, too bad'.[5] Although Downing Street quickly rejected these allegations, the suspicion remains that old people are seen by some in government as a disposable liability. According to Dr Mike Ryan, the executive director of the World Health Organization's health emergencies programme, herd immunity is a dangerous concept; he warns that the use of this term 'can lead to a very brutal arithmetic which does not put people and life and suffering at the centre of that equation'.[6]

'Harvesting' is a term used in epidemiology to capture a temporary increase in mortality rates above and beyond normal expectations, although this is not a term used in public, for obvious reasons. The excess mortality rate caused by an environmental phenomenon such as a heatwave is a standard example of 'harvesting'. There is reason to believe that some politicians in the UK embraced the notion of harvesting, though not as an inevitable natural consequence. Instead, harvesting became an acceptable direct consequence of government policy. Richard Coker, Emeritus Professor of Public Health at the London School of Hygiene and Tropical Medicine, makes a persuasive argument that the UK government's initial strategy was herd immunity and harvesting: 'the initial strategy of allowing herd immunity to develop in the wider community was pursued, but the most vulnerable people were not protected. Though harvesting may not have been the government's intention, it became the de facto policy in the absence of adequate protections for older and vulnerable people.'[7] Care homes took the full force of this epidemiological tsunami.

In most countries the majority of fatalities from COVID-19 related illnesses have occurred in nursing and care homes, not hospitals. In Ireland the figure is 63 per cent, and we can assume that something similar is true across Europe. The fact that for the first few months of the pandemic the UK government only reported deaths in hospitals but not in nursing and care homes was not only a deceitful way of massaging the numbers to make things look less disastrous than they were, but also a sign of disrespect for those who passed away in isolation in care homes: in the UK these deaths don't seem to count, literally. It is now beyond doubt that in the preparations most countries made for the pandemic, nursing and care homes were not a priority, as reflected by the mortality rates.

In the UK the Office for National Statistics reported 17,422 deaths of care home residents from COVID-19 between the end of March and 5 June 2020, accounting for 47 per cent of the total number of deaths caused by the virus; the fact that infected hospital patients were allowed to return to care homes, even though they had tested positive for COVID-19, and the lack of access to testing and personal protective equipment in care homes, were two significant contributing factors.[8]

In Ireland, the UK, and across Europe thousands of people lost their lives prematurely because care homes lacked the protective equipment and financial resources to cope with the coronavirus outbreak. Society's relationship to people living in old age has never been under closer scrutiny. This is why there has never been a better time to go back 2,000 years to a philosophical work by Marcus Tullius Cicero, *Cato the Elder on Old Age* (44 BCE).

Cicero on old age

In this text, one of the earliest philosophical explorations of old age, Cicero defends the counter-intuitive view that old age is arguably the best part of one's life, hence refuting the generally held prejudice against people in old age as weak, vulnerable, helpless, and dependent, incapable of making meaningful contributions, and thus a mere burden to society.

Cicero considers, and refutes, four standard reasons why old age is considered to be undesirable. First, we are told that old age is bad because it makes us unproductive. Cicero refutes this assumption on the grounds that in old age, while we may not be as physically strong as in our youth, we are wiser, and that this is infinitely more important: 'Great deeds are not done by strength or speed or physique: they are the products of thought, and character, and judgment. And far from diminishing, such qualities actually increase with age.'[9]

Second, it is said that old age is bad because as we get older we get physically weaker. Cicero dismisses the implications of this argument. Of course one is physically stronger in youth, but physical strength is less important than intellectual ability, which improves with age: 'Every stage of life has its own characteristics: boys are feeble, youths in their prime are aggressive, middle-aged men are dignified, old people are mature.'[10]

Third, the prejudice against old age is, partly, a consequence of our over-sexualized society. Old age is looked down upon because we fear that it deprives us of almost all sexual pleasures. Cicero considers this but dismisses it as nonsense. First of all because, contrary to what the younger generations think, people in old age still have sexual desires and are sexually active. But even if old age flattens our libido, according to Cicero this is only to be welcomed, since old age gives us freedom from a type of slavery: 'I have known many old men who had no complaints about their age or its *liberating* release from physical pleasure.'[11] Why liberating? Because in youth reason is, and always will be, the slave of sexual passions. Desires of a sexual nature obstruct one's reasoning and muddle one's intelligence, or as Cicero says: 'let sensuality be present, and a good life becomes impossible'.[12]

Fourth, old age is assumed to be bad because it is not far removed from death. We touched on this issue in the Introduction, and as we know, Cicero thinks that this is a non-starter: following in the footsteps of the Epicurean philosopher Lucretius, Cicero is adamant that death is not something we should fear.

Admittedly Cicero's paean to old age is not without blemishes. One issue is the fact that 'old age' is a notoriously nebulous concept. Small children think that anyone over 30 is 'old', and over 40 'very old'. What Cicero referred to as old age is very different from what we consider to be old age. Compared to our Roman ancestors today the threshold of old age has shifted by about twenty years, so much so that human life, traditionally divided into three stages, has been extended to the so-called 'fourth age'.

Also, Cicero was writing for a class of people who would naturally have had many slaves to look after them in old age, which is very convenient; we can only speculate how Cicero would have felt about coping with the challenges of old age, from restricted mobility to incontinence, without slaves to look after him. Be that as it may, we have much to learn from Cicero. There are many aspects of Cicero's analysis that are still as valid today as they were 2,000 years ago. Having refuted four standard arguments as to why old age is bad, Cicero argues that it is to be welcomed, not scorned: it is in old age that we are most productive intellectually, which is the most valuable type of work. The problem is that society fails to recognize the contribution that people can still make in old age, and this is potentially a great injustice.

A matter of respect

The received view today is that 'old age' starts when people reach retirement, around the age of 65 (allowing for national variations). The dividing line between young and old is drawn when a person is deemed to be no longer economically productive, no longer able to make a meaningful contribution to society: people in old age are 'over the hill' or 'past their sell-by date' or 'has-beens'. And to the extent that our society shows concern for people in old age, it is only because, deep down, we pity them for being more vulnerable, more weak, more ill, less autonomous.

We need to resist this misconception of old age, just as Cicero did many years ago. He reminds us that we should not pity people for being old; instead we should recognize the fact that people in old age still have a great deal to offer to society, that old age does not make us useless or worthless. Modern society has ceased to see its senior citizens as citizens; instead it considers them as a burden, both financially and morally. The reason why society today looks down on old age will be addressed below, when we explore the dominant role of autonomy in modern conceptions of morality.

Today, as we try to come to terms with the most devastating public health crisis in a century, many older doctors are giving up the comfort of their retirement, putting on the scrubs and joining in the herculean effort in the front line, saving lives in hospitals around the world, while putting their own lives at risk in the process. Anthony Fauci, who is 79, has been the director of the National Institute of Allergy and Infectious Diseases (NIAID) in the US since 1984, and has served under eight presidents. He is a key figure in the Trump administration's White House Coronavirus Task Force that is addressing the pandemic, although he has been sidelined by Trump for daring to contradict the president on the best way to deal with this crisis.[13] On 19 October 2020, a few weeks before the presidential election, Trump attacked the nation's top infectious disease expert as a 'disaster', adding that 'people are tired of hearing Fauci and all these idiots'.[14]

At the same time, many of us living in lockdown at home have enjoyed the fruits of the labour of people in old age, reading novels by Margaret Atwood or John le Carré, watching Patrick Stewart or Judi Dench on the small screen, or listening to the Rolling Stones performing via Zoom as part of the 'One World: Together at Home' concert. And it goes without saying that most philosophers are like good Chianti: they get better with age. Martha Nussbaum was 71 when she published *The Monarchy of Fear* (2018), Bernard Williams was 73 when he published *Truth and Truthfulness* (2001), and Onora O'Neill was 74 when she published *Constructing Authorities: Reason, Politics, and Interpretation in Kant's Philosophy* (2015).[15] On a personal note, I like to think that my best work is yet to come.

Of course, it is not all about those who are famous or established. We should value all older adults as the guardians of historical living memory, the gatekeepers of our bygone personal identity, and our unique, living connection with the past. Unfortunately, since memories are intangible from a monetary perspective, these things are not always valued by modern society.

Autonomy and old age

In the previous chapter the point was made that to make sense of social injustice we must think in structural terms, not just in terms of individual acts of injustice. COVID-19 has exposed the way that, at an institutional level, those in old age are not always treated with the same concern and respect as other people in society. Modern society tends to look down on people who lack autonomy, and by implication it looks down on old age. By gradually losing their autonomy people in old age also lose their moral status, and society feels legitimized in treating them as second-class citizens. This raises the question of whether autonomy should be the gold standard in our moral universe.

Autonomy is not an easy concept to define. There are two ways to think about autonomy: as a property that characterizes an individual person, or as something that applies to groups. Both are considered highly valuable, but it is best to consider them separately. The idea of group autonomy is much older than individual autonomy; in fact it was from the notion of group autonomy that the modern fixation with individual autonomy matured. An example of a group seeking or claiming autonomy would be a nation. As a group concept, it is the political goal or aspiration for autonomy from dominant alien powers that is behind the secessionist dreams of separatists in Catalonia today, as it was in Ireland before 1921, and as it has been of every other nation that has fought and does fight against colonial powers. For these groups, autonomy is a fundamental prerequisite of freedom, where freedom is defined as the absence of domination by external sources.

It was from the idea of autonomous nations that in seventeenth-century Europe we moved to the idea of autonomous individuals. If nations can be autonomous, why can't we, as individuals, also claim our autonomy? But in making this switch, from groups to individuals, the idea of autonomy also changed. When we say that a person is autonomous, or has autonomy, we don't mean simply that this person is not under the dominion of others. What we mean is something different: when applied to individuals, autonomy refers to a set of diverse qualities, entitlements, or characteristics, including self-governance, liberty rights, privacy, individual choice, liberty to follow one's will, and being one's own person.

As individuals we value autonomy because it allows us to express our own unique sense of identity. Autonomy stands for self-determination, or self-rule, which we value for a simple but powerful reason: it is a statement of the fact that this is me, this is my life, and I'm in control of it. All this in part explains why the concept of autonomy has a positive connotation: we think of autonomy as something desirable and indispensable, and of the opposite of autonomy as harmful, even shameful.

I'll say more about the opposite of autonomy in a moment, but first, why are we so well-disposed towards autonomy? In *The Morality of Freedom* contemporary philosopher Joseph Raz defines autonomy in terms of 'being the author of one's own life' and 'the vision of people controlling their own destiny'.[16] The case for autonomy seems very strong: who doesn't want to be the author of one's own life? Who doesn't want to control one's own destiny? This is exhilarating stuff. It's invigorating. Autonomy gives us a purpose, and that's precisely why we value it.

And there is more. It is not simply autonomy that we value, but we also value the fact that others show respect for our autonomy. To respect a person's autonomy is, first, to recognize that person's capacities and perspective, including her right to hold views, to make choices, and to take actions based on personal values and beliefs. In fact, respect encompasses even more. It demands treating others so as to allow or enable them to act autonomously. It could be said, therefore, that true respect is an action: the act of respecting others, not the mere adoption of a certain attitude.

For all these reasons autonomy is generally considered a powerful and benign moral concept, which seems to have no downsides. This makes it curious that this idea of autonomy, as an individual virtue, was not always recognized as an important moral principle. It is only in the last 300 years that autonomy has become a central preoccupation in moral theory. In the history of Western philosophy this is referred to as the invention of autonomy, as J. B. Schneewind argues in his outstanding work of that title.[17] And the philosopher almost unanimously credited for this invention is Immanuel Kant. What is distinctive about Kant's contribution is not simply that he draws our attention to autonomy as a moral concept, but that he thinks that autonomy is the core concept of morality; with Kant, we have a full theory of morality as autonomy.

Kantian autonomy presupposes that we are rational agents. Rationality makes it possible for us to control our desires. It is through rationality that we become responsible for our actions, and that responsibility is fundamentally what morality is about. So, in Kant's morality as autonomy, rationality cannot be separated from autonomy, or in other words, autonomy is intrinsically linked to our power to reason. We are free to the extent that we have the power to reason. It is because of our autonomy that we are, from a moral point of view, equal. Autonomy belongs to every individual. Autonomy is our moral compass. Our moral capacities are made known to each of us by the fact of reason, which we can use against the pull of desire.

Kant argued that respect for autonomy flows from the recognition that all persons have unconditional worth, each having the capacity to determine his or her own destiny. It is for this reason that Kant suggested that autonomy is closely related to dignity. To lose our autonomy is to lose our dignity.

To recap, autonomy started as a concept that applied to groups, in particular nations. It then moved to being a concept that applies to each and every individual. It then became a moral concept, and finally, it became almost synonymous with morality.

This is all very interesting, and perhaps evidence of progress in our collective moral thinking. It would seem impossible not to define a moral person independently of their individual autonomy. But what does this say about old age, and the gradually receding autonomy that people experience as they approach the final stage of their lives? Autonomy may not be as benign as we think.

Dependency and interdependency

Could it be that autonomy has a less attractive side? In other words, is the Kantian idea of morality as autonomy overrated? Yes, perhaps. It is beyond question that when we, as individuals, assert our autonomy, we are expressing an ideal that is highly individualistic. To declare one's autonomy is to remind others that we can go it alone, that we don't need help from anyone, that we are self-sufficient. In direct opposition to what John Donne said in his famous sermon in 1624, autonomy proclaims that every man and woman *is* an island, entire of itself.

At one level this is a very attractive ideal, for all the reasons we have already given. But like many ideals, it is not a reality, at least not for everyone. And so, what happens if someone does not have autonomy, because they cannot be autonomous? How are we to engage, morally speaking, with someone who does not have the faculty or capacity of autonomy? And remember, that 'someone' could be anyone, you or I included.

There is more to autonomy than the narrow, reason-based conception favoured by Kant. People can lack autonomy for any number of different reasons. In some cases, the person may have never developed the means of acting autonomously, for physical or mental reasons. A person might be born with a physical or mental disability that prevents them from being self-sufficient. That person will always struggle to be autonomous, and perhaps will never be able to be autonomous. In other cases we find that a person can possess autonomy at a certain point in their life, but lose that autonomy at a later stage. This might be the result of an accident which causes an immediate, radical change in one's life, for example a head injury caused by a car accident; or it might be a slow process that takes a person in their old age to a position where they are no longer self-sufficient.

Whatever the reason why a person is not, or is no longer, autonomous, the question is: if we define our morality in terms of our autonomy, what does that say about people who have never been autonomous? Or what happens, morally, to a person when they lose their autonomy? Does losing one's autonomy mean losing our moral standing? This seems to be what Dominic Cummings thinks.

I believe there are three risks associated with autonomy that we need to consider. First, not being autonomous might make someone feel morally inadequate, since without our autonomy we are made to feel like a lesser moral person. Secondly, lacking autonomy can make one feel like a burden to others. Being a drain on others can be interpreted in terms of being a nuisance, because we need others to help us get on with our day-to-day lives, but it can also be interpreted as being a moral burden: you impose your needs on others who, as a result, are under a moral duty to assist you. Thirdly, lacking autonomy means that we have become a burden to society. Instead of making a valuable contribution to the common good, we become a net cost, a weight that others have to bear.

This is the ugly side of autonomy, or to be more precise the ugly side of a morality defined in terms of autonomy. This is also something that people in our hyper-individualistic, productivity-obsessed society don't like to talk about. But talk about it we must. One way to think about the limits of the moral appeal of

44

autonomy is to think of the antithesis of autonomy. According to binary logic, if autonomy is good, the opposite of autonomy must be bad. But what is the opposite of autonomy, and is it bad? Most textbooks of philosophy will tell you that the opposite of autonomy (ruling oneself) is heteronomy (being ruled by others). Heteronomy is obviously bad, since no one wants to be ruled by others. Being under the domination of others is the antithesis of being free, as the philosophers of the civic republican tradition, from Marcus Tullius Cicero in the first century BCE to Quentin Skinner and Philip Pettit in the twentieth and twenty-first centuries, have told us.

But it's not as simple as that. I want to suggest that there is a different concept that captures the opposite of autonomy: it is not heteronomy, but 'dependency'. The concept of dependency has both negative and positive connotations, but it is the negative aspects that dominate our collective imagination, while the positive ones are neglected and often forgotten. When, for example, we think of drug addiction as a physiological dependence on narcotic substances, dependence is synonymous with self-enforced slavery, which is neither desirable nor enviable. However, I think it is imprudent, and unwise, to think of human dependency exclusively as something bad, something to be avoided. If we started from a different assumption, namely that dependency is an inescapable feature of the human condition, then it wouldn't be considered good or bad; it just is. And it is wrong to think of dependency as an exceptional circumstance. The way to think about dependency is that it is merely a reminder of our intrinsic vulnerability, and it is this vulnerability that makes human interconnectedness intelligible. As the philosopher Judith Butler points out, we cannot understand bodily vulnerability outside of a specific conception of relations, since the body is defined by the relations that make its own life and action possible.[18] Butler is right to remind us that we can only be human inasmuch as we are vulnerable to each other, and that we don't pre-exist our vulnerability. What is required is a paradigmatic shift in our conceptual framework from dependency to interdependency. This would allow us to value the centrality of dependency and interdependency in human relations. Interdependency speaks to a sense of community and solidarity that is lost in the moral preoccupation with autonomy in modern society.

Of course, it's extremely hard to embrace interdependency today, in our modern capitalist society, precisely because the ideal of individualism and individual autonomy reigns supreme and is not to be challenged. In her book *Love's Labor* Eva Kittay talks about what she calls the 'dependency critique' of the ideal of equality, where she takes issue with autonomy in particular: 'The dependency critique is a feminist critique of equality that asserts: A conception of society viewed as an association of equals masks inequitable dependencies, those of infancy and childhood, old age, illness and disability.'[19] What we can learn from Kittay's radical contribution to moral and political philosophy is that autonomy is at best an ideal, at worst a myth. We find a similar message in two other important studies: Martha Albertson Fineman's *The Autonomy Myth: A Theory of Dependency* puts an emphasis on those who care for dependants, while Adriana Cavarero's *Inclinations: A Critique of Rectitude* reminds us that the liberal individualist model of the independent self is a 'mirage', or in other words that invulnerability is an invention.[20]

Philosophers tell us that there are different degrees of autonomy. I think that's the wrong way to think about the human condition: there are only different degrees of interdependency. The ideal of autonomy has many virtues, but excessive autonomy can also be a vice. And while morality as autonomy is a very alluring ideal, this way of thinking about morality risks overshadowing other important moral considerations: dependency, interconnectedness, an ethics of care, solidarity, community, hospitality, perhaps even love.

Conclusion

Modern society treats people in old age according to the principle of social justice as reciprocity: fairness demands that those who have given to society in the productive part of their lives should receive back from society in the later, unproductive stage of their lives. The anxiety and apprehension we project on to people

in old age is well intended, but it may also do a dis-
service to the people it wants to benefit. In particular,
the assumption that being old and being unproductive are synonymous is misguided and potentially
insulting.

As the COVID-19 pandemic radically reshapes the
face of our society, we must ensure that one of the
lasting changes it brings lies in the way society relates
to those living in old age. The COVID-19 crisis has
demonstrated that there is an urgent need to shift away
from the model of care in nursing homes to alternative approaches that enable older people to live well in
their own homes. We cannot afford to let COVID-19
set the clock back.

The fact that in the first few months of 2020 so
many people in old age died in care homes is shameful,
and reflects a laissez-faire attitude towards this group
in our society that is morally disturbing. Our conde-
scending and patronizing view of the elderly will have
to be revisited. We must find a way to reverse society's
tendency to feel pity for those in old age because their
autonomy is slipping away. One important lesson we
must learn from this pandemic is that old age is not
regrettable and undesirable; instead it is the ideal of
autonomy, and in particular the morality of autonomy,
that is fundamentally problematic.

The justification for cocooning the elderly during
the present public health crisis should not have been
on the grounds that they are vulnerable or weak, but
because they are precious, and they still have a lot to

give. As Cicero said: 'To be respected is the crowning glory of old age.'[21] This pandemic has fully exposed the lack of respect our efficiency-obsessed modern society has for people in old age.

4

Life under lockdown:
nasty, brutish, and short?

> On the whole men are more good than bad; that, how-
> ever, isn't the real point. But they are more or less igno-
> rant, and it is this that we call vice or virtue; the most
> incorrigible vice being that of an ignorance which fan-
> cies it knows everything and therefore claims for itself
> the right to kill.
>
> Albert Camus, *The Plague*.

The potentially devastating impact of COVID-19 on the
world economy is beyond the scope of measure. UN
Secretary General António Guterres has expressed concern that the pandemic could trigger conflicts around
the world.[1] The heart-warming pictures of Italians sing-
ing from their balconies at the start of the crisis were
gradually replaced by mounting incidents of social
unrest, with increasingly longer queues at food banks.
As national lockdowns during the first wave of the pandemic are being replaced by local lockdowns to combat
the second wave, there is a growing fear that this could
lead to civil disorder. While the first lockdown restrictions were perceived, overall, to be fair, in part because
people felt that we were 'all in it together', reimposing

selective restrictive measures will be perceived differently. Social psychologist Clifford Stott fears that because local lockdowns will be far more likely to fall on disadvantaged and ethnically mixed communities, they will aggravate and amplify existing inequalities and social tensions, with the serious risk of undermining social cohesion and provoking civil disorder.[2] In the UK, Leicester was the first place to go into local lockdown at the end of June 2020, and went into local lockdown again in early September. In October 2020 Manchester was forced into lockdown, against its will, and without adequate financial support from central government. Andy Burnham, mayor of Greater Manchester, declared that the restrictions were certain to increase levels of poverty, homelessness, and hardship.[3]

There is also the added risk that if the economy collapses it will bring down civil society with it.[4] Political philosophers have a term for this: we are being propelled towards the 'state of nature'; and depending on one's conception of the state of nature, this is not necessarily a good thing.

This chapter will suggest that while disaster might bring out the best in children, in part because they have a natural belief in a better world (as novelist Anne Enright has argued in her reflections on the lockdown), it is also the case that an extreme crisis tends not to bring out the best in adults.[5] During the weeks of lockdown there was a worldwide surge in domestic violence, with António Guterres going as far as to say: 'I urge all governments to put women's safety first as they respond to the pandemic.' In Latin America things were particularly bad: in El Salvador between March and April 2020 there was a 70 per cent increase in reports of domestic violence compared to 2019; in Colombia there was a 51 per cent increase; in Venezuela there was a 65 per cent increase in femicide in April compared to a year earlier; and in Honduras the number of reported cases of domestic and intra-family violence increased by 4.1 per cent per week from the start of the pandemic.[6] Domestic violence, the other pandemic associated with coronavirus, will be discussed in more detail in Chapter 8.

This chapter will explore the pessimistic, almost nightmarish account of the state of nature, which has a long tradition in the history of philosophy. At the centre of it we inevitably find the widely maligned but often misunderstood seventeenth-century English philosopher Thomas Hobbes. At the risk of defending a highly controversial figure, not generally loved by the left because of his support for an all-powerful authoritarian figure at the centre of the polity, I want to suggest that Hobbes still has a great deal to teach us, especially about life under COVID-19.

Hobbes and the plague

It is a little-known fact that Hobbes was not unfamiliar with life during a plague. Hobbes died in 1679, thirteen years after the Great Plague of London, which lasted from February 1665 to 1666; 100,000 Londoners died from the Black Death, or one-fifth of the population. But even aside from the Black Death, plagues were a recurring event, ever-present in Europe between 1346 and 1671. France lost almost a million people to the plague in the epidemic of 1628–31. That was after the plague of 1585, which killed 14,000 people in Bordeaux alone, about a third of the population: the mayor of Bordeaux at the time was Michel de Montaigne, the philosopher we met in the Introduction.[7]

This historical fact explains a minor detail in the famous illustration for Hobbes's 1651 masterpiece *Leviathan*, designed by engraver Abraham Bosse, but with creative input from Hobbes himself (Fig. 1).[8] In this iconic image we find at the forefront the figure of the sovereign king, whose body is literally and figuratively constituted by the amassing of individual bodies: these are the co-signers of the social contract, the creators of the modern sovereign, an artificial person built up from the consent of the multitude. As Hobbes explains: 'A multitude of men, are made one person, when they are by one man, or one person, represented; so that it be done with the consent of every one of that multitude in particular.'[9]

The Leviathan towers over a landscape and a city. The city is almost completely deserted, with only a few figures walking its streets. And there are two odd-looking minuscule figures, with something over their heads. A closer look at these two figures reveals that they are, in fact, plague doctors, with their characteristic beaked masks containing herbs or sponges soaked

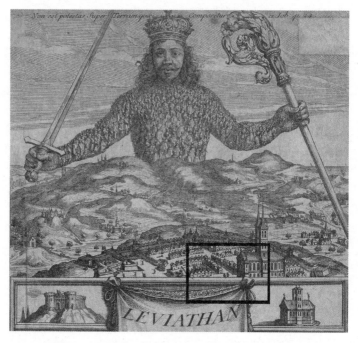

Figure 1 Engraved title page of the first edition of
Leviathan (1651)

in vinegar to filter the air (Fig. 2). This apparently
minor detail is significant for at least two reasons.
First, it tells us that Hobbes was more familiar than
we are with living with infectious diseases. Secondly,
he understood that the primary motivation behind
creating a stable political society is the fear of death.
In other words, our world in 2020 has a lot more in
common with Hobbes's world in 1651 than we think,
and perhaps there are still things we can learn today
from this seventeenth-century philosopher.

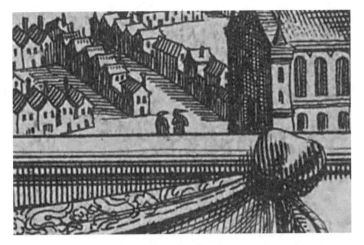

Figure 2 Detail from the title page of *Leviathan* showing plague doctors

The state of nature

Of course, Hobbes is not famous because of his views on the plague, but for introducing the powerfully evocative concept of the 'state of nature'. Contrary to what is often assumed, the state of nature for Hobbes is only a hypothetical construct which he introduced to explain and justify the essence of civil society, and in particular the nature and scope of the modern state. In his text Hobbes makes it very clear that the state of nature was not an archaic state of affairs that actually occurred in the remoteness of the past; instead it is something that can occur at any moment, and that we must guard ourselves from. Whenever political authority breaks down, it is replaced by the anarchy of the state of nature.

Anarchism is one of the most important and original traditions in political philosophy, and deserves to be taken seriously. Grounding their beliefs in a systematic theory of non-hierarchical social organization, the philosophers of anarchism advocated non-violence and equality;[10] anarchist ecology is still today a vibrant school of thought which enjoys a long and distinguished tradition, counting Henry David Thoreau and Leo Tolstoy among its early champions.[11] In terms of COVID-19, it has even been suggested that when central authority fails in performing socially crucial tasks – as it has in the US, judging from the inadequate response to the pandemic[12] – informal networks and civil society organizations step up and perform the tasks of the central authority. In the UK there have been many cases of fundraising initiatives for the benefit of the National Health Service, including Margaret Payne, from Ardvar, Sutherland, who raised £75,000 by climbing the equivalent of Mount Suliven (2,398 ft) on her stairs at home, and army veteran Captain Tom Moore, who completed 100 laps of his garden before his 100th birthday to help raise money for NHS Charities Together. Captain Moore originally pledged to raise £1,000 but has since received more than £33m in donations. These instances of mutual aid, solidarity, and grassroots organization vindicate the perennial appeal of anarchism.

Hobbes, who lived through the English Civil War (1642–51), had other ideas about anarchy. For him, the state of nature was not a pretty place:

> In such condition, there is no place for Industry;
> because the fruit thereof is uncertain; and consequently
> no Culture of the Earth; no Navigation, nor use of the
> commodities that may be imported by Sea; no commo-
> dious Building; no Instruments of moving.[13]

A few months into COVID-19 the world did not regress
completely into a Hobbesian state of nature, but there
were alarming indications of it. As lockdown measures
were enforced on every society across the globe, we didn't
anticipate the experience of, in the words of Hobbes, 'no
account of Time; no Arts; no Letters; no Society'; as I
write these pages there are still no theatres, no concerts,
no travel, and no sporting events. There are no weddings
and no funerals. As lockdown measures were extended
for longer, we also started to see initial manifestations
of what Hobbes called the 'war of all against all': countries aggressively outbidding each other on the global
market for coronavirus protective equipment;[14] the US
buying virtually all the stocks of a drug proven to work
against COVID-19, leaving the rest of the world with
nothing for three months;[15] and anti-lockdown protests
in the US, including heavily armed rallies enjoying the
blessing of President Trump.[16] According to estimates
from a firearms analytics company, Americans bought
nearly 17m guns in the first ten months of 2020, more
than in any other single year. The political response of
Trump to COVID-19 will come under closer scrutiny in
Chapters 5 and 6.

Hobbes goes on to capture the essence of the state of
nature in chilling and memorable terms: 'And which

is worst of all, continual fear, and danger of violent death; And the life of man, solitary, poor, nasty, brutish, and short.'[17] COVID-19 has instilled fear in all of us – continual fear. Initially people made fun of the fear that toilet paper might run out, but behind the laughter there was the serious fear that anyone and everyone could find themselves at death's door.

Fortunately, Hobbes also teaches us that we are not doomed, that it is possible to escape the state of nature. The only way to survive the state of nature is via cooperation, which is the essence of the social contract. For all its misery and wretchedness, the state of nature is also a state of equality. In the state of nature we are all mortal and vulnerable. That is certainly true of life under COVID-19. This virus does not distinguish between nationalities or ethnicities, gender or social class, religion or language, even though as we have seen in Chapter 2, COVID-19 strikes hardest where there is inequality and poverty, as reflected by the class and race divide in the death rates. Nevertheless, today we are all at risk, and from this fundamental equality another reality ascends: only unity, trust, teamwork, and solidarity will keep COVID-19 at bay.

To escape the Hobbesian state of nature we need to forge a new social contract: a mutually beneficial agreement where everyone agrees to make sacrifices in the short run on the understanding that everyone will be better off because of it in the long run. Similarly, to overcome COVID-19 we will need to commit to an unprecedented level of sacrifice, trust, and social cooperation. Living under temporary lockdown and maintaining physical distancing is a big sacrifice for many people, especially as unemployment escalates and many businesses are on their knees, but we must have trust in the World Health Organization and in our public health experts (*pace* Trump), since these emergency measures will work only if everyone complies without exception. Non-hierarchical 'horizontal' organizations at the grassroots level can do a lot of good in difficult times, and this was certainly the case in the early months of the pandemic, but when a crisis is as severe and far-reaching as what we are facing today, it can only be overcome by unanimous cooperation, and enforcing this necessitates a central authority.

The fool

Mutual social cooperation is fragile and tentative at the best of times, especially in a capitalist world where selfishness is a virtue and greed rewarded. The biggest threat to social cooperation is the self-serving actions of free-riders who want to benefit from people's spirit of cooperation without doing their bit for the common good. Hobbes had a term for this type of person: *the fool*.

As Hobbes explains, the fool believes that there is no such thing as justice, and that it is legitimate to break a contract in the pursuit of self-interest. The world is full of fools, and it is in times of crisis that their true nature is fully exposed. At the start of the pandemic we encountered them in supermarkets panic buying, and as lockdown restrictions ease we find them in public areas refusing to adhere to safe measures of social distancing. They run businesses that exploit people's fear by overcharging for food, face masks or hand sanitizers. And then there are those politicians whose muddled reaction to the coronavirus crisis will not be forgotten, especially by the families of the people who died because of their incompetence. These include Brazil's far-right president Jair Bolsonaro, who continues to downplay the pandemic, notwithstanding the deaths of 162,000 people, which makes Brazil the third worst country in the world for deaths and infections. Mexico's president Andrés Manuel López Obrador openly ignored the advice of public health officials, shaking hands with his supporters, kissing their children, and joking that he was relying on good-luck charms – religious images, four-leaf clovers, and a $2 bill he carries for good luck – to protect him during the crisis.[18] There is also Donald Trump, who initially dismissed coronavirus as a hoax, wasting precious life-saving time, and Boris Johnson in the UK, who dragged his feet over enforcing the same restrictions on movement as the rest of Europe; Dominic Cummings as well, whose initial response was to endorse an absurd but deadly policy of herd immunity. And we must not forget Anders Tegnell, the state epidemiologist of the Public Health Agency of Sweden, which has the eighth highest number of coronavirus-related deaths per capita in the world. On 23 October

2020 Sweden registered 1,870 new coronavirus cases, the highest since the start of the pandemic. On the same day Norway registered only 193 new cases.

These are the fools who, according to Hobbes, will face their comeuppance. By failing to adhere to the norms of social cooperation they will only succeed in establishing their reputation as unreliable, imprudent, and untrustworthy, and for this they will be ostracized after we leave the state of nature and re-establish the normality of civil society.

Hobbes misunderstood

Fiction is a powerful force in shaping social understanding. It can also have immense impact on political modelling and philosophical analysis. From Plato's allegory of the cave to Margaret Atwood's *The Handmaid's Tale*, via Jonathan Swift's *Gulliver's Travels* and Voltaire's *Candide*, the dividing line between fiction and philosophy has always been very thin.

In the early part of the twentieth century a number of novels shaped philosophical discourse, not always for the better: Aldous Huxley's *Brave New World* (1932) and Ayn Rand's *Atlas Shrugged* (1957) come to mind. And then there was William Golding's *Lord of the Flies* (1954), a novel that makes us despair for the human condition. Golding's novel has often been read as a fictionalized account of the Hobbesian state of nature.

Rutger Bregman's book *Humankind* refuses to accept the Hobbesian conclusions one might draw from reading Golding's novel.[19] The subtitle of Bregman's book summarizes his thesis in three words: *A Hopeful History*. In this book he challenges the dystopian scenario in Golding's novel by reminding us of a little-known real-life case from 1966 of six boys stranded on a deserted island south of Tonga in the Pacific for more than a year. Their experience was nothing like that of *Lord of the Flies*: they survived because they lived in harmony, cooperating with one another, helping each other. For Bregman this story is an invigorating endorsement of everything that is good and noble about human nature, contrary to what Hobbes (and Golding) seem to assume. In philosophical terms, Bregman sides with Jean-Jacques Rousseau against Hobbes on the state of nature: a much more benign place, grounded in a more positive conception of human nature.[20]

As a philosopher, Bregman's story leaves me cold. In terms of theorizing human nature we have to take what we read in a novel with a pinch of salt, and similarly we cannot and should not draw any conclusions about human nature from one case study, fascinating as it undoubtedly is. In other real-life contexts of scarcity, people have been known to turn to cannibalism. In a famous case from 1884, a four-man crew sailing from England to Australia were shipwrecked with almost no food. When the 17-year-old cabin boy became ill, two of the men decided to kill and eat him. After being rescued, the two men were convicted of murder and sentenced to death – later commuted to six months' imprisonment. We can only speculate what the six boys on the island in the Pacific Ocean would have done if they had run out of food, and had not been rescued after a year; but whatever might have happened, I would certainly not draw any conclusions from it in terms of the essence of human nature.

What is interesting about Bregman's analysis is that, not for the first time, Thomas Hobbes is portrayed as the bogeyman of political philosophy. Bregman rejects the well-known Hobbesian view of the state of nature, according to which, without a society to restrain our most basic instincts, people left to their own devices will turn on each other, and society will collapse into an abysmal anarchy, a 'war of all against all', where life is solitary, poor, nasty, brutish, and short. This seems to be the message of *Lord of the Flies*. The real-life case of the six boys from Tonga is Bregman's way of telling us that Hobbes was wrong. Furthermore, Bregman rejects the vindication of authoritarianism often associated with Hobbes's political theory. On both counts I believe Hobbes is being misunderstood.

First, Hobbes is accused of reducing human nature to the most base, ugly, evil mindset: selfishness. This is an erroneous reading of his work. It is true that self-interest plays a dominant role in Hobbes's political theory, but it is wrong to correlate self-interest with selfishness, just as it is wrong to assume that self-interest is synonymous with greed or avarice. Scottish Enlightenment philosopher David Hume (1711–76) argued that if certain conditions did not obtain, justice would not be advantageous. These conditions, which

Hume called 'circumstances of justice', include moderate scarcity, moderate selfishness, and equality. As Hume famously said: 'It is only from the selfishness and confined generosity of men, along with the scanty provision nature has made for his wants, that justice derives its origin.'[21] The point being that we must be realistic about politics: self-interest will not go away just because we don't like it. We must find ways to confine its most destructive tendencies, not pretend that it does not exist.

Let us remember that plague was part of the historical backdrop at the time Hobbes was writing. This means that fear, and fear of death in particular, was part of the historical context, not to mention the civil war that prompted him to write *Leviathan*. It is true that Hobbes assumed that people will act in their own self-interest, but self-interest here does not mean greed or selfishness, merely the desire to stay alive. I cannot disagree with Hobbes on this point; in fact I doubt anyone can disagree with him. The same desire to stay alive is what is behind our daily actions now that we are learning to live with coronavirus. If I wash my hands, self-isolate, keep social distancing, and wear a mask in public places, as I do, it's because I fear death and it is in my interest to stick to these rules. Of course I also do those things so as not to inflict death on others, in case I'm a carrier of COVID-19. Keeping the virus under control, restricting its spread, and being able to go back to theatres, concerts, restaurants, and to see and hug our loved ones is in everyone's self-interest.

Hobbes never said that human nature is evil, but only that our main and greatest motivation is to avoid death, and we appeal to our self-interest to stay alive. He also says that, by nature, we are blessed with 'prudence', which he defined as foresight, grounded in experience: 'Prudence is but experience, which equal time equally bestows on all men, in all things they equally apply themselves unto.'[22] Reading about the six boys living for a year on a desert island only reinforced my view that Hobbes was right: thanks to prudence they soon realized that the best way for them to survive was by working together, cooperating, helping each other out. And prudence is also behind all the recommendations of the scientific community on how to cope with and defeat COVID-19.

Crucially, good things can come out of our self-interest. During a pandemic, the best way to stay alive, and what is ultimately in our self-interest, is via social cooperation. This is the genius of Hobbes: he is arguably the greatest thinker of mutually beneficial social cooperation, because he doesn't ground cooperation in altruism but in self-interest.

The other reason why Hobbes is widely disliked is because in 1651 he argued that the only way out of the state of nature is via the formation of an all-powerful sovereign, the *Leviathan*, depicted in the frontispiece of his book. Since then, Hobbes has been accused of justifying authoritarian dictatorship. This anachronistic reading of Hobbes is misleading and unhelpful.

The figure of the Leviathan is easily misunderstood. The issue here is not whether one prefers an authoritarian dictatorship to a democracy, but instead whether it is best to organize political life under one central authority as opposed to no authority at all. Hobbes's political theory addresses the latter case. All Hobbes is saying is that it is in our interest to organize social and political life under the protection of a central authority, which, in the words of Max Weber, successfully claims the monopoly of the legitimate use of force within a territory. Weber here has given us the most famous and succinct definition of the modern state.[23]

Hobbes was not a fascist, he was merely a statist. Of course, there are very good reasons why one might be sceptical about the invention of the modern state, but as I will argue in the concluding chapter of this book, there are times when we ought to be glad that our political affairs are planned by a modern state. In particular, during a pandemic crisis the cooperation that is needed cannot be left to the spontaneous actions of individuals, but needs to be coordinated, and that requires orchestration from the top. Social cooperation, and perhaps society more generally, is an artificial social construct, not a natural certainty.

Conclusion

Philosophers have been pondering the true essence of the state of nature for centuries, and this debate is not going to be settled any time soon. While advances in social psychology and neuroscience give us new perspectives on this question, we will not find the answer in science. Some questions are, and always will be, of a strictly philosophical nature.

Hobbes is criticized and maligned for assuming that humans are quintessentially evil, but this is a misreading of his political theory. What he is telling us is that we should not start from the assumption that we are naturally good and well disposed towards one another; instead it is the context that determines how we behave. In a state of nature, where we fear for our lives, we are driven by self-preservation to do anything in our power to stay alive. And that includes being nasty towards our fellow human beings, or as Hobbes puts it: 'And because the condition of man … is a condition of war of everyone against everyone … it followeth that in such condition every man has a right to everything, even to one another's body.'[24]

The COVID-19 crisis has brought out the best and the worst in people. Writing in *The Irish Times*, Joe Humphreys wants us to believe that people are mainly good, and the outpouring of neighbourliness, solidarity, and self-sacrifice during the lockdown is just another marker of that fundamental truth.[25] There is some truth in this, but at the other extreme we have seen a frightening increase in domestic violence worldwide during the lockdown period.

Just as in Hobbes's state of nature, living with COVID-19 is a reminder of the emancipatory politics of social cooperation, but we cannot assume that this will occur spontaneously. We are entering the territory of a new social contract, which will form the cornerstone of a new civil society post COVID-19. We need to bring back the state, to reclaim the idea of the common good, and above all to repossess the territory that neoliberalism handed to the profit-maximizing private sphere on a golden plate.

5

Is COVID-19 bad for populism?

> The evil that is in the world always comes of ignorance,
> and good intentions may do as much harm as malevo-
> lence, if they lack understanding.
>
> > Albert Camus, *The Plague.*

Before we had COVID-19 we had populism. Until
recently the popularity of Boris Johnson and Nigel
Farage in the UK, Matteo Salvini in Italy, and Marine
Le Pen in France was unequivocal, but almost insignificant compared to that of Jarosław Kaczyński in
Poland and Viktor Orbán in Hungary. And that's only
in Europe. Modern-day populism is founded on a specific but crude and somewhat distorted understanding of the social and political landscape, where the
excluded masses are oppressed by a ruling elite.

Populist movements are the self-proclaimed dissent-
ing political forces out to shatter the status quo. An
irreverent, nonconformist agenda explains populism's
attraction, especially right-wing populism, which is
the subject of this chapter. By giving a voice to the
powerless, the populists' aspiration is to dislodge
the ingrained interests of the power-elite. Populism is

the voice of the excluded against the entrenched elite; their leaders see themselves as the re-embodiment of Saint George slaying the elitist dragon, or David defeating Goliath. But the COVID-19 pandemic may have exposed the underlying weakness and long-term inadequacy for effective political leadership of core populist positions. This chapter will start with an analysis of populism: what it is, why it has been so successful electorally, and what this success tells us about modern democracy.[1] This will be followed by considerations of the potential impact of the COVID-19 crisis on populism. In particular, I will argue that populism might turn out to be one of the most illustrious fatalities of this crisis.

Populism explained

Prone to simplistic analysis, the complex phenomenon of populism is often dismissed as a transitory episode, a fleeting blip that will wane as quickly as it has appeared. This is a mistake: right-wing populism is here to stay, unless its menace is countered. What is at stake is not simply the revival of an intolerant, regressive, divisive, right-wing political ideology, but the collapse of the politics of toleration, and with it potentially the unravelling of the European project.

Taking a leaf from Cas Mudde's extensive work, two aspects of modern-day populism can be highlighted: first, that it is not just a mentality or a proclivity, but a political ideology, with clear policy implications.[2]

Secondly, that populism is founded on a specific but crude and somewhat distorted understanding of the social and political landscape where only two political groupings exist: the perfidious, corrupt elite, holders of the reins of political and economic power, and the excluded masses, 'the pure people'.[3] This appraisal of social dynamics, constructed around a simple dichotomy, has a long history. The Romans organized their affairs around two mutually exclusive social ranks, patricians and plebeians, and two centuries ago Marx diagnosed the world of capitalism as consisting of two main classes, the bourgeoisie and the proletariat. This binary stance is still prevalent today in the collective social imagination, with many colourful formulations in our current modern jargon: the rich and the poor; us and the 'other'; the haves and the have-nots.

Among scholars of populism there is a debate about whether, and to what extent, populism poses a threat to democracy. Influential scholars such as Nadia Urbinati are adamant that populism is the antithesis of democracy,[4] although others argue that populism is not per se anti-democratic; instead populism is only incompatible with *liberal* democracy. As William Galston explains: 'the aim of contemporary populism is what many scholars and at least one national leader (Orbán) call "illiberal democracy" ... From this perspective, populism is a threat not to democracy per se but rather to the dominant liberal variant of democracy.'[5] Liberal democracy is a type of indirect, representative democracy. What make this type of democracy liberal is the

assumption that good government is grounded on freedom of thought (including religious toleration), freedom of expression (especially freedom of the press),
and equal citizenship rights, regardless of class, race,
or gender. In a liberal democracy, individuals exercise
their autonomy through regular elections, and political
parties compete for people's votes.

The tension between populism and liberal democracy is also highlighted by Daniele Archibugi and Marco
Cellini, who argue that in spite of analytical differences, populism originates from the general discomfort
with the inability of *liberal* democracies to fulfil their
promises.[6] This viewpoint seems obvious, even innoc-
uous. By juxtaposing populism and liberal democracy,
Archibugi and Cellini are following a long tradition
in contemporary political theory. Margaret Canovan,
one of the most insightful scholars of populism, claims
that modern liberal democracy is an uneasy combina-
tion of two fundamentally different sets of principles:
liberal on the one hand (concerned with individual
rights, universal principles, and the rule of law) and
populist/democratic on the other (the sovereign will of
the people, typically expressed through referendums).
This is what she refers to as 'the two-strand theory of
democracy' at the heart of liberal democracy.[7]

One potential problem with analysing populism
through the prism of the two-strand theory of democracy is that it gives the impression that populism is
only as old as liberal democracies, which is misleading; populism predates liberal democracy by many

centuries. Similarly, reading Galston, Archibugi, and Cellini, one gets the impression that populism is somehow intrinsically related to the liberal interpretation of democracy we have become accustomed to in the West over recent times. Again this is misleading, and it may even distort and misrepresent certain key aspects of populism.

In a nutshell, the issue is this: populism cannot be defined as a challenge to *liberal* democracies since populism has been around a very long time, and it predates liberal democracies by many centuries. Populism is much older than Locke, Hobbes, or John Stuart Mill. In fact, looking at ancient forms of populism can be both instructive and revealing, since it can help us have a better understanding of the contemporary phenomenon of populism, especially in Europe.

Populism: old and new

I suggest we go back to Ancient Rome, and the last years of the Republic. Consider the case of Publius Clodius Pulcher, better known simply as Clodius, one of Ancient Rome's best-loved bad boys. He was a social rascal and a political radical, scandalously promiscuous and libertine. Gaining notoriety in 62 BCE when he gatecrashed a solemn, all-female religious festival, he then became one of the most violent and politically dangerous leaders of a populist faction that engineered the exile from Rome of the most ardent defender of the Republic: Cicero. Clodius went on to terrorize the streets of Rome with his private militia. But apart from using violent means to shake the foundations of the status quo, his political project also included radical reforms in the interests of the common people, the Roman plebs, including passing laws that made the distribution of grain in the city entirely free.

There is one curious aspect of Clodius's life that makes his political biography compelling and of particular interest to anyone studying populism today: Clodius was born to a rich, powerful, established, patrician family. What he did in order to gain political power was both unprecedented and remarkable. He turned his back on the patrician roots of his family and asked to be adopted by a plebeian family. As the inimitable Mary Beard puts it: '[Clodius] has gone down in history as the mad patrician who not only arranged to be adopted into a plebeian family in order to stand for the tribunate but also put two fingers up to the whole process by choosing an adoptive father younger than himself.'[8]

In an innovative, non-monarchical political system defined by a complex balancing act between an elite of senators of conservative disposition, hell-bent on maintaining the status quo with all the privileges it bestowed to the small number of ruling families, and a growing underclass of plebeian citizens who had some political representation through the appointment of official tribunes of the people (*tribuni plebis*), the populist card was often used in the years of the Roman

Republic to press on with radical political reforms, often accompanied by bloodbaths.

Of course, populism was not invented by Clodius. Before Clodius brought mayhem to Rome, the long shadow of populism was cast by two legendary brothers, Tiberius and Gaius Gracchus, who both served as tribunes of the people in the late second century BCE. Their political agendas and methods were distinctly populist. One brother attempted to pass land reform legislation that would redistribute the major aristocratic landholdings among the urban poor and veterans; the other brother pushed for a subsidized quantity of grain for each citizen of Rome. Both were assassinated for their political vision.

The parallels between the Gracchi brothers and Clodius are many, including the fact that although the Gracchi brothers were officially plebeians, they were born into the old and noble Sempronia family. Their father held all the major political offices in the Republic: tribune of the plebs, praetor, consul, and censor. Their mother was a patrician, Cornelia Africana, daughter of Scipio Africanus, a hero of the war against Carthage.

What can Clodius and the Gracchi brothers teach us about populism in the twenty-first century? One thing above all: contrary to what is generally believed, populism is not a bottom-up political movement, the desperate voice of the marginalized masses, the political expression of a final, radical, democratic push by those who for too long have been excluded, and are not going to take it any longer. Instead, populism is the brainchild of the elite; it is much more of a top-down phenomenon than we are led to believe. That's how it was in Ancient Rome, and that's how it is today.

Just like 2,000 years ago, populism today arises in the context of a clash between different factions of the ruling elites: it is the articulation of a calculated political strategy used by one sector of the elite in order to gain the upper hand over another sector of the elite. In the last analysis, populism can be explained in terms of the masses being manipulated by some members of the elite, for the interest of the latter only. Seen in this light, populism is a tried and tested political strategy, much older than liberal democracy. Where Clodius and the Gracchi brothers failed, Julius Caesar succeeded: born into a powerful and privileged family, Caesar's populist appeal was instrumental to undermining the rule of law, culminating in his appointment as 'dictator for life'.

Archibugi and Cellini suggest conceptualizing populism in terms of differences between 'incumbents' (elites) and 'new entrants' (excluded masses) in the political arena. I think they are right, but only partially. Yes, it is correct to conceptualize populism in terms of incumbents and new entrants, but it is wrong to assume that the new entrants are the excluded masses. Instead, we should think of the new entrants as part of the elite, to be precise that part of the elite that is excluded by another part of the same elite from holding the reins of power.[9]

Just as in Ancient Rome, modern leaders of right-wing populist movements almost always emerge from privileged backgrounds. Donald Trump positioned himself as the saviour of the white, marginalized American lower classes, notwithstanding his family's status among America's wealthiest elite. He may speak the language of modern-day American plebeians, claiming to be the champion of the underclass, but he was never one of them. The same is true of Nigel Farage in the UK. A founding member of the xenophobic UK Independence Party (UKIP), Farage sold Brexit to the British people by siding with the British working class against the interference of the European Union in British affairs, and the growing threat from immigrants to British jobs. But Farage was educated at a fee-paying private school, and his father was a stockbroker who worked in the prestigious financial district in the City of London. Farage's predisposition to be seen drinking pints of beer in a pub is equivalent to Trump's red baseball cap: symbolism and props can go a long way towards pretending to be what one is not. Trump and Farage, like Caesar and Publius Clodius Pulcher before them, had to shrug off their elitist social class in order to champion the interests of the masses.

The perpetual appeal of populism today

Generalizations about populism in politics are always hazardous. Nevertheless, the lexicon of the modern populists reveals two recurring themes: anti-intellectualism and provocation.

Anti-intellectualism can be defined in terms of the denigration, even ridicule, of intellectual pursuits. It also includes, in the words of Colleen Shogan, 'a rejection of the elitism and self-aware attitude of distinction that is commonly associated with intellectual life'.[10] Because populist leaders want to identify with the masses, they portray intellectuals as the high-brow end of the elitist faction, and predictably direct their scorn towards the literati, journalists, artists, and especially academics. The closure of the Central European University in Budapest perfectly follows this script. Donald Trump has made anti-intellectualism his own personal mantra.[11] In a series of interviews Trump said that he doesn't need to read extensively because he has the gift of making the right decisions 'with very little knowledge other than the knowledge I [already] had, plus the words "common sense", because I have a lot of common sense and I have a lot of business ability'. This in part explains why he believes that he instinctively knows what is the right thing to do – 'A lot of people said, "Man, he was more accurate than guys who have studied it all the time"'[12] – and why he thinks that reading long documents is a waste of time. Not surprisingly, Trump is also sceptical of experts, since as he says, 'they can't see the forest for the trees'; we will return to the question of experts in Chapter 7.

Anti-intellectualism is also the reason leaders of populist movements gravitate towards provocation in their political rhetoric. They tend to communicate via a direct and often vulgar prose, deriding political correctness, and regularly infringing norms of respectful verbal interaction. During his successful presidential campaign, Jair Bolsonaro recommended that parents should beat their effeminate boys, and that he would prefer a dead son to a homosexual one.[13] Like Bolsonaro, Trump is also a master at this type of political rhetoric. In politics the gains to be had from using belligerent, toxic, divisive language can be considerable. And populists have no qualms about sacrificing truth if it brings them votes, as we will discuss in the next chapter.

COVID-19 and populism

The global COVID-19 crisis is unprecedented, although it was not unexpected. It is the biggest social, political, and economic challenge the world has faced since the end of the Second World War. Whether this crisis will strengthen or abate the rise of populism is something worth considering; it was after the economic shock of the First World War and the 1918 flu pandemic that Europe put its trust in far-right populist solutions, and with millions of jobs wiped out almost overnight by this pandemic the prospect of history repeating itself is not as far-fetched as it may sound.

The populist response to this crisis has been as swift as it was predictable. Microbiology was given a racial makeover when Donald Trump kept referring to COVID-19 as the 'Chinese virus' or 'Kung flu', blaming the crisis not on a submicroscopic infectious agent but on the non-white 'other'. And in Hungary, Viktor Orbán made sure that no good crisis should go to waste by sucking the last few remnants of democracy out of the Hungarian political system, duly closing down parliament and concentrating even more power in his own hands.

Regarding the pandemic's impact on populist politics more broadly, one possible scenario, put forward by Cas Mudde in a piece published in *The Guardian*, is that while it might kill hundreds of thousands of people worldwide, we should not expect it to 'kill populism'. The reason for this is that 'populism' does not have one, unitary response to the pandemic: 'In short, there is not one single "populist response" to the coronavirus pandemic. There is not even a single "rightwing populist response". Populist parties and politicians have responded very differently, in part depending upon whether they are in government or opposition.' As Mudde says, this crisis will have at best a moderate overall effect on populists: some will win, some will lose, and some will stay the same.[14]

The view that populism will not come out badly from this crisis, and may even come out stronger, is defended by three other prominent political scientists: Allan Stam, Paulina Ochoa Espejo, and Rogers Brubaker. Stam highlights the fact that younger generations are bearing the economic and social costs of the economic downturn caused by the lockdown far more than their more senior counterparts, a fact that may dramatically increase the appeal of national populism for these prospective voters. In the US, right-wing populists will want to shift the costs to those whose health is most at risk in order to protect the employment prospects of the economically productive generations, particularly those in the suburbs and manufacturing areas. Populist leaders can use their framing of the 'American way of life' to fuel support for populist policies. Trump has done this, with some success.[15]

Ochoa Espejo fears that even the pandemic will slide off populism's Teflon coating. The Teflon politician effect, as she calls it, shows that voters do not focus on the validity or soundness of a politician's arguments or policies. This Teflon-coated quality of populist leadership comes from two sources: first, a style of political discourse and personal action aimed at keeping followers continuously mobilized; second, a strategy of deploying the core followers' support as a smokescreen to cover the destruction of institutions from within.[16]

Other populist world leaders have adopted the same tactics that worked for Trump. This has been true during the pandemic, regardless of how each leader has reacted to the crisis. Like Trump, Mexico's Andrés Manuel López Obrador pretended at first that nothing was going on. Brazil's Jair Bolsonaro called it 'a little flu'. In Hungary, Viktor Orbán used the coronavirus emergency to pass a law that allows him to rule by decree indefinitely. Recep Tayyip Erdogan in Turkey has used the crisis to increase authoritarianism. In India, a brutal lockdown that was instituted within hours of its announcement did nothing to diminish Narendra Modi's popularity. Rodrigo Duterte of the Philippines has enforced the toughest measures during the lockdown, even claiming that those who disobey will be shot dead, but his supporters still approve of his management of the pandemic. In sum, it seems that the tolerance of unacceptable behaviour in populist politicians is a global trend.

Arguing along the same lines as Stam and Ochoa Espejo, Brubaker points to the fact that although the pandemic has not generated a coherent populist response, it has created a reservoir of popular anger, which has 'heightened distrust of expertise, exacerbated antipathy to intrusive government regulation, and amplified skepticism toward elite overprotectiveness'.[17]

These are all strong arguments suggesting that COVID-19 will not harm populism, and if anything might even make it stronger. There is, however, a different scenario that ought to be considered. It is possible that COVID-19 might have exposed the soft underbelly of populist politics. To be precise, there are at least three areas where populism might come out badly from this crisis. First, if we have learned anything from the last few months, it must be that unity and not division will see us through. Our racial, national, and religious divisions, exacerbated by populists for their own electoral gains, have become insignificant: no one with moral integrity should dare to resent the immigrant nurses, doctors, and hospital cleaners heroically working in our health services, risking their lives on a daily basis. Suddenly Brexit seems like a daft idea.

Secondly, in times of crisis people look for and demand skilful leadership, not bombastic jokers. The difference between Jacinda Ardern and Boris Johnson is immeasurable. In the US four years of a joke president has been long enough.[18] What might be amusing in normal times, and even electorally beneficial, becomes toxic in hard times. The COVID-19 crisis is baring every political naïvety and inadequacy, every incompetence and ineptitude. Few politicians will come out unscathed from this, but many populist politicians will be seen to have been wanting in their most basic job requirements. At a time when indecision costs lives, everyone is being reminded that politics is too important to be left in the hands of the unscrupulous, the unprincipled, and the opportunistic. Our necessary reliance on highly skilled experts during the current crisis reveals the idiocy of populism's anti-intellectualism: never before have university professors and their research been so valued and respected.

Bolsonaro's affirmation that the experts are wrong and that this pandemic is nothing more than a hoax will not be forgotten;[19] nor will Xi Jingping's duplicitous denials nor Trump's meddling and muddling.[20] Many minor politicians are already being punished by voters for their opportunism. In New Zealand, in a desperate attempt to hold on to power, Jami-Lee Ross, MP for the centre-right National Party, played the COVID-denier card by siding with the 'plandemic'

movement. Plandemic refers to a pair of 2020 con-
spiracy theory videos which promote falsehoods and
misinformation about the COVID-19 pandemic. This
was a huge political gamble that went badly wrong.
Not only did Ross perform disastrously in the October
2020 national election won by Jacinda Ardern's
Labour Party, but in a post-election TV interview he
was torn to pieces by Tova O'Brien, political editor for
Newshub. The video clip of her telling him 'I don't
want to hear any of that rubbish' went viral on social
media platforms.[21]

There are already signs that we are seeing the beginning of the end of populist politics. Danielle Allen,
head of Harvard's Safra Center for Ethics, believes
that this moment is nothing less than an 'existen-
tial crisis' that will reshape American society. As
she explains: 'The democracies led by populists – the
U.S., the United Kingdom, Brazil – have done poorly,
and the democracies led by institutionalists have
done well.'[22] In November 2020 Donald Trump lost
the presidential election to Joe Biden, which will be a
severe blow to populists all over the world. The ripple
effects of Trump's failure to secure a second term in
the White House will be felt globally. Trump's defeat
could trigger a domino effect that will make right-
wing populism even less attractive to many more
countries. There is also growing evidence to suggest
that support for populist beliefs in Europe has fallen
markedly over the past year. A survey carried out by
the YouGov–Cambridge Globalism Project, based on

26,000 people in 25 countries, shows a considerable decline in populist tendencies in 2020.[23]

Finally, in Europe at least, populist movements always side with nationalist sentiment to the detriment of the European Union. This position may be untenable post-crisis. COVID-19 has demonstrated the inability of national economies to deal with this crisis. Instead it has shown how a concerted effort of all European nations, led by the European Central Bank and the many instruments at its disposal, is the best and only hope for a swift recovery. What the citizens of Europe need going forward is a stronger EU, albeit one with a sturdier socialist agenda.

It will take many years to recover from this crisis. Politically the situation is volatile, and anything is possible, but this scenario is not beyond the realm of political reality: it sees populism coming out much weaker than before, as a peripheral and almost negligible ideology on the political landscape. Similarly, right-wing neoliberal politics is likely to be reassessed in favour of a stronger state-run economy, with a nationalized health service at its core, including in the United States.

Conclusion: the end of populism?

This chapter has defended a position that is slowly but consistently gaining support from some influential scholars of populism: namely, that COVID-19 could inflict a major blow to populism.[24] Time will tell who is right, but a word of caution: even if it turns out that COVID-19 punishes populism, as I predict, this doesn't mean that populism will disappear. Populism is as old as democracy itself, and as long as there is democratic politics, there will be populism.

6

COVID-19, fake news, and post-truth

There always comes a time in history when the person who dares to say that $2 + 2 = 4$ is punished by death
Albert Camus, *The Plague*

In crises, we rely desperately on the truth, and there is no room for 'post-truth'. Or at least, there shouldn't be. But that's not what we have seen with the COVID-19 pandemic. In the previous chapter we saw how populism tends to have a relaxed relationship with truth. In this chapter, the focus will switch to the phenomenon of fake news and post-truth, and how COVID-19 is not immune from this aspect of the global populist trend.

Lies are part of the DNA of modern society, though we often now refer to them with the more dignified terminology of marketing, advertising, propaganda, or spin. From unscrupulous sellers of used cars to prime ministers making unsubstantiated declarations about weapons of mass destruction, it seems that many people today make a living from lies. And of course there is also the growing industry responsible for generating fake news on every social networking platform on the

internet. In the public imagination politicians are pro-
fessional liars *par excellence*, or as the writer George
Orwell once put it: 'political language is designed to
make lies sound truthful and murder respectable, and
to give an appearance of solidity to pure wind'.[1]

This chapter will start by distinguishing between
lies and post-truth, before highlighting the subversive
nature of post-truth, and how not even something as
serious as COVID-19 is immune from the rhetoric of
post-truth.

Lies, damned lies, and post-truth

In 2016 'post-truth' was declared the 'Word of the Year'
by Oxford Dictionaries. The prefix 'post' in post-truth
is crucial to an accurate understanding of this concept.
There is a fundamental difference between concepts
such as 'post-natal' or 'post-surgery', and other concepts such as 'post-sexuality' and 'post-truth'.[2] The
'post' in the former group indicates a chronologi-
cal sequence, a moment after a specified situation
or event. The concepts in the latter group, including post-truth, are different; here the prefix refers to
a time in which the specified idea has become redundant and can therefore be safely discarded. As Oxford
Dictionaries explains, rather than simply referring to
the time after a specified situation or event – as in
post-war or post-match – the prefix in post-truth has
a meaning more like 'belonging to a time in which
the specified concept has become unimportant or

irrelevant'. The prefix 'post' in post-truth is there to indicate that 'truth' is no longer essential, that it has become obsolete, and has been superseded by a new reality.

The Oxford English Dictionary gives the following definition of post-truth: 'an adjective defined as relating to or denoting circumstances in which objective facts are less influential in shaping public opinion than appeals to emotion and personal belief'. This definition is not incorrect, but there is more to post-truth than it suggests. The OED definition centres on the subjective nature of post-truth in contrast to the objective nature of truth, which is potentially misleading. While subjectivism is an important feature of post-truth, this is not necessarily its primary or distinctive characteristic. In order to see what makes post-truth a disturbing political concept, it is necessary to distinguish post-truth from a mere lie.

Consider the following statements by two recent American presidents. The first is Donald Trump's tweet on 6 November 2012: 'The concept of global warming was created by and for the Chinese in order to make U.S. manufacturing non-competitive.' The second is Bill Clinton's testimony on 26 January 1998: 'I want to say one thing to the American people, I want you to listen to me, I'm going to say again, I did not have sexual relations with that woman, Miss Lewinsky.'[3]

Clinton's statement, given the subsequent revelations, is alarming. It is possible that by appealing to a technicality Clinton did not consider his intimate interactions with Monica Lewinsky as 'sexual relations', but that is unlikely; it would require a phenomenal effort of self-deception or ingenuity to defend that position with honesty and integrity. Trump's tweet is also disquieting, but for different reasons. While both Trump and Clinton are, to use modern slang, 'messing with the truth', there is a fundamental difference between these two presidential proclamations. Clinton told a lie, while Trump's statement is a paradigmatic example of post-truth. The point about telling a lie is that the liar accepts that there is a truth, knows what the truth is, but decides to tell a different story. In an odd way the liar honours the truth by denying it. Trump's case is radically different. He is dismissing truth, making truth redundant, superfluous. This is what post-truth does: it doesn't simply deny or question certain facts, instead it aims to undermine the theoretical infrastructure that allows us to assess the evidence that points to the truth.

When Trump writes in a tweet (28 January 2014): 'give me clean, beautiful and healthy air – not the same old climate change (global warming) bullshit! I am tired of hearing this nonsense', he is saying that what has been established on scientific grounds is merely 'bullshit'. This is what post-truth looks like: it is a deliberate attempt to delegitimize scientific findings and research. Trump is threatened by the evidence of climate change, therefore he dismisses climate change by denying the evidence.

I'm going to suggest the following definition of post-truth, which is different from the definition we find in the OED: *Post-truth is a deliberate strategy aimed at creating an environment where objective facts have little influence in shaping public opinion, where theoretical frameworks are undermined in order to make it impossible to have a rational, evidence-based discussion that aims at uncovering the truth, and where scientific truth is delegitimized.*[4]

Post-truth in the twenty-first century

Notwithstanding its present-day popularity, there is in fact nothing new about the concept of post-truth. Trump did not invent post-truth, he is merely the boldest, loudest present-day embodiment of this phenomenon. In its earlier incarnations it overlaps with some interpretations of scepticism, nihilism, or simply rhetoric, which suggests that the idea of post-truth is as old as philosophy itself.

In her essay 'Truth and Politics', originally published in *The New Yorker* on 25 February 1967, Hannah Arendt was already lamenting the fact that politics and truth don't mix. Arendt distinguishes between political lies in the pre-modern and the modern world. The pre-modern traditional lie had two distinguishing qualities: first, it was never meant to deceive literally everybody; it was only meant to deceive the enemy. Secondly, the traditional lie concerned only particulars facts, or in the words of Arendt, 'tears in the fabric of factuality'. The modern lie, in contrast, allowed no last refuge for the truth, since the liar deceived himself as well. Moreover, the modern lie was no longer a tear in the fabric of reality; instead, because modern political lies are so extensive, they require a complete rearrangement of the whole factual texture, the making of another reality.[5]

When referring to modern political lies, Arendt had in mind twentieth-century totalitarian ideologies, which she accused of being seamless reconstructions of reality. Even though Arendt writes about 'modern political lies', what she is saying is a better description of post-truth than a lie; but of course Arendt didn't have that terminology at her disposal in the 1960s. Perhaps the only difference between the modern political lies of totalitarian regimes and post-truth today is the fact that post-truth is a political phenomenon that occurs also in *liberal* democracies, and is not an exclusive resource of totalitarian regimes. Liberal democracies might *reduce* the risk of post-truth, which is why we might be surprised when post-truth surfaces in them, but it would be naive to assume that they *eliminate* the risks of post-truth. The notion of 'truth' has not always enjoyed uncontested approval and universal endorsement, not even in liberal democracies.

There is an obvious explanation for the present preoccupation with post-truth, which I will, however, refute: namely, it has everything to do with one person, since never before has post-truth enjoyed the support of the President of the United States. For the first time, the legitimization of post-truth is coming from the top, to be precise, from the White House. We are accustomed to political leaders establishing 'the truth'; the old adage that history is written by the victors goes a long way towards explaining this phenomenon. Today we are faced with the scenario, at times surreal, of someone who holds the highest political position in one of the most powerful nations in the world showing contempt for the truth.

Donald Trump's relationship with truth is disconcerting and dangerous. For the last four years Trump's incessant accusations of fake news against the main media outlets, including the *Washington Post*, the *New York Times*, and CNN, has reflected a longstanding disdain for the truth. Unlike other politicians who, at times, try to deny certain facts, Trump is determined to undermine the theoretical infrastructure that makes it possible to have a conversation about the truth. His strategy is to create an environment where objective facts are less influential than they ought to be in shaping public opinion, where the theoretical frameworks necessary to make sense of certain events are scorned.

While Trump undoubtedly has a lot to do with the current obsession with post-truth, to suggest that he created an entirely new political phenomenon is to give him too much credit. It is unhelpful, and misleading, to focus exclusively on Trump; it would be a mistake to give him more power or influence than he already has. So while Trump may have taken this phenomenon to a new level, post-truth is not new; it was not 'made in America'.

Post-truth and the fear of truth

Hannah Arendt, one of the most astute political thinkers of the twentieth century, was undoubtedly right to warn us that it is the nature of the political realm to be at war with truth, in all its forms. That is because, as Arendt says, 'truth carries within itself an element of coercion'.[6] This is a powerful statement, worth reflecting on. What Arendt is telling us here is that anyone in power will do anything to resist truth, since truth has a 'despotic' character: there can only be one truth, and truth does not bend to political pressure or coercion. This is why truth is hated by tyrants, since they rightly fear the competition of a coercive force they cannot monopolize.

The abhorrence of truth, and in particular its coercive nature, goes some way towards explaining Trump's attorney Rudolph W. Giuliani's remarkable claim that 'truth is relative'. This was said in the context of special counsel Robert Mueller's request for an interview with Trump regarding the Russia investigation. Giuliani raised concerns that Trump could perjure himself because 'truth isn't truth'. He then went on to explain that 'They may have a different version of the truth than we do.' This is further confirmation, if any was needed, that post-truth today is a phenomenon that starts from the very top, that consensus on post-truth can be manufactured, and therefore that consensus cannot always be trusted to produce the best argument.

Post-truth is an invention of the powerful, not the powerless. It comes from the top, specifically with the intent to undermine the truth. The distinctive feature of the phenomenon of post-truth is that it uses the arsenals of truth against truth itself; its aim is to establish a new consensus around post-truth in order to weaken the old consensus around truth. This is where the paradox lies: post-truth appropriates the notion of consensus, central to the literature on truth, in order to undermine the consensus around truth and in the process legitimize the idea of post-truth.

COVID-19 and fake news

The COVID-19 crisis was seen by Trump and his administration as another opportunity to undermine scientific truth. By questioning the wisdom of the experts in the World Health Organization, or by insinuating that this virus was created in a Chinese laboratory, or by dismissing the pandemic as a mere hoax, Trump did his best to delegitimize scientific truth. Trump interpreted the disagreement between experts as a damning condemnation of scientific knowledge and advice; the topic of experts' disagreement will be the subject of Chapter 7.

This is the major difference between a lie and post-truth. While a lie subverts a specific truth, post-truth tries to subvert truth itself. Post-truth is much more devious and dangerous to the democratic fabric of our society than a lie. We can cope with politicians lying – at least liars are sensitive to the truth, and they are not always very good at covering their tracks – but in this crisis we cannot afford the risk of allowing politicians to delegitimize truth.

Since the start of the pandemic the science of coronavirus has been repeatedly challenged, to such an extent that it is becoming increasingly hard to know who to believe and who not to believe. Some politicians, especially those sympathetic to right-wing populist tendencies, made up all sorts of stories about the virus, blurring the line between scientific truth and post-truth. Trump was quick off the mark, at first dismissing COVID-19 as a hoax, and subsequently blaming the Chinese for the cataclysm. Trump referred to COVID-19 as 'the Chinese virus', and later as 'Kung flu', and even hinted that the virus originated in a lab in Wuhan, even though there is no evidence of this.[7]

At the end of September 2020 the US registered 7.5 million cases of COVID-19 (roughly one-fifth of all confirmed cases worldwide) and 210,000 deaths. As the number of infections and deaths in the US surpassed the worst projections, the spotlight moved to Trump's ill-advised comments on how to treat the virus. Following his bizarre suggestion that coronavirus might be treated by injecting disinfectant into the body,[8] the Centers for Disease Control and Prevention published a survey which showed that 39 per cent of 502 respondents reported engaging in non-recommended, high-risk practices, including using bleach on food, applying household cleaning or disinfectant products to their skin, and inhaling or ingesting such products. Twenty-five per cent of the adults contacted in this survey suffered from at least one adverse health effect as a result of harmful practices.[9] Trump also suggested irradiating patients' bodies with UV light, an absurd idea quickly dismissed by doctors.

Each time Trump made a wild recommendation on how to deal with COVID-19, he was undermining the legitimacy of the scientific community. This is the essence of post-truth. Although he did not inject himself with disinfectant, he admitted to taking the anti-malaria drug hydroxychloroquine for over a week to prevent coronavirus infection, even though this is not a recommended or proven treatment.[10] In fact, clinical trials showed that hydroxychloroquine had no benefit for patients hospitalized with COVID-19. The fact that Trump's beliefs regarding hydroxychloroquine as a treatment for COVID-19 lack any scientific backing has not stopped Bolsonaro in Brazil from endorsing it, and the Ministry of Health in Brazil even issued new guidelines on its use.[11]

Some recommendations

Like populism, post-truth will never go away. It is wishful thinking to hope that it will spontaneously retreat and disappear, never to be seen again. If there is room for truth in our scientific and social discourse, there will always be someone prepared to promote post-truth.

Arendt said that truth is hated by tyrants because they fear the competition of a coercive force they cannot monopolize. She is right, but only in part. It is more accurate to say that truth is hated by (almost) all politicians, not just tyrants. Liberal democracies thrive on disagreement and conflict. Where there is no disagreement there lies dictatorship, but where there is disagreement there is the potential for multiple consensuses, including a consensus for post-truth. The topic of disagreement in the scientific community will be the subject of the next chapter, but what can be done about post-truth? How do we respond to this menace? Given that post-truth is here to stay, the challenge is to be ready for it when it raises its head, and to have mechanisms in place to combat it.

Post-truth can be fought on two separate fronts: the institutional and the personal. At the institutional level the threat of post-truth can be alleviated in two ways. First, via the consolidation of checks and balances in a mixed constitution between the three main branches of government: executive, legislative, and judiciary. In recent years we have witnessed an increasing attack on the separation of the different branches of government from unscrupulous politicians who believe that those who hold the reins of executive power have the right to exercise control over the judiciary. Recent developments in Hungary, for example, suggest that Viktor

Orbán is trying to limit judicial independence by restricting the freedom of judges to interpret the law, posing a serious threat to the rule of law. Any threat to the constitutional separation of powers must be resisted and fought, without reservations and restraint. For example, Hungary's ruling Fidesz party should be expelled from the European Peoples Party (EPP), and perhaps Hungary from the EU.

Secondly, the threat of post-truth can be alleviated at the institutional level by reinforcing the 'fourth' branch of government: the media. It is imperative that newspapers and other channels of information remain independent from the executive branch of government, and their impartiality fully protected. Measures need to be put in place that will prevent any one person or syndicate having control over the distribution of information by having a monopoly or disproportionate influence over mass media outlets. But that's not all. The concept of 'mediatization' captures the phenomenon whereby the media increasingly influences and penetrates various social spheres, including the political sphere. Perception and knowledge of politics become increasingly mediatized, and their distinctive boundaries increasingly blurred. The problem is not only that technological innovation, and smartphones in particular, have made it possible for media consumption to be immediate and ubiquitous, but that media content has become highly personalized. What is different and unique about politics today, compared to the past, is the fact that today we live in a world where there is total deregulation of both the formation of, and access to, information. The internet has made consensus on post-truth much easier to manufacture, and as we know, when political knowledge and entertainment mix, post-truth flourishes.[12] According to a study published in the journal *Nature: Human Behavior*, Facebook spreads fake news faster than any other social website, faster than Google or Twitter.[13] Tighter legislation on social networks is long overdue, redefining their legal identity as 'publishers' rather than mere 'platforms'.[14]

At the personal level, work can be done on the area where epistemology overlaps with ethics. Here it is necessary to accept our own personal responsibility regarding the proliferation of post-truth. Media outlets are not the only culpable parties in the explosion of post-truth: consumers of information also bear a moral responsibility. There is a tradition in the history of Western political thought, originating in the work of John Locke, according to which citizens in a liberal society have a duty to do their best to hold beliefs that are true or very likely to be true. This duty has sometimes been called the 'alethic obligation', from the Greek term for truth, *aletheia* (ἀλήθεια).[15] If we accept our alethic obligation, then our responsibilities as believers increase rather than diminish. This is in stark contrast to the prophets of post-truth, who want to release us from our alethic obligations.

Conclusion

It is hard to see silver linings in these dark times. Hundreds of thousands of people have lost their lives, and many survivors are still struggling to make a full recovery. But in the last chapter it was argued that perhaps populism as a global ideology might come out of this crisis weaker than it was at the end of 2019; and given that populist leaders have a tendency to propel ideas of post-truth, one potentially positive outcome of this crisis is that truth will regain its value while post-truth will be, if not dismissed, at least treated with much more caution.

Over the last few years the politicians of post-truth, many of them right-wing populists, have declared war on impartial, fact-based news outlets, with considerable success. This world crisis might put a stop to that, to the benefit of these fact-based news outlets and all of us who still have trust in science and the pursuit of truth.[16]

Misinformation is dangerous at the best of times, but potentially lethal in times of crisis. The highly deregulated virtual economy of search engines and social media platforms might also become one of the victims of this pandemic: Facebook, Google, and many other social platforms are going to be with us for a long time yet, but they are starting to change the way they operate, and making an effort to counter fake news, and that can only be a good thing.

Writing in *Psychology Today*, Chrysalis L. Wright is right to warn that fake news regarding COVID-19 is spreading almost as fast as the virus itself, but while some social media platforms are now taking measures to remove fake news and misinformation from their platforms, 'it is ultimately up to us, as consumers, to make sure that the information we are feeding ourselves is accurate, factual, non-biased, reliable, and true'.[17] We can fight fake news, and post-truth, and populism, but to do so we have to face up to our individual responsibilities.

7

COVID-19, experts, and trust

Stupidity has a knack of getting its way; as we should see if we were not always so much wrapped up in ourselves.

Albert Camus, *The Plague*

In times of crisis, the norm is to do what the experts tell us. In times of health crisis, listening to public health experts, and acting accordingly, becomes a rational and ethical imperative. After the outbreak of the most serious public health emergency in living memory, governments around the world are making decisions based on advice from public health experts, and all of us 'ordinary' citizens are told to listen to this advice and follow their directives. So far so easy, but it gets more complicated.

Across the world businesses have shut down, university campuses have closed, sporting and cultural activities have ceased. In places where there used to be music, laughter, and chatter there is now only the sound of silence. No weddings, no funerals. In Europe, the UK and Sweden initially dragged their feet, but have since aligned with the international consensus.

In both countries, the reluctance to take early, decisive action was bordering on the criminal; in the UK Neil Ferguson, former scientific adviser to Boris Johnson, said that the number of coronavirus deaths in the UK could have been halved if the government had introduced the lockdown a week earlier.[1] This is appalling but not surprising; about 150,000 people attended the horse racing festival at Cheltenham on 16–19 March, only a few days before lockdown measures began, something that was met with a mix of incredulity and alarm. What is even more disconcerting is that in allowing the Cheltenham festival to proceed the British government was standing behind the advice of its medical chiefs, even though this advice was radically different from the experts' advice to other governments around the world.

Knowledge and trust

There are good epistemic and moral reasons for following the advice of the experts: most of us don't have their knowledge and experience, we don't have time to acquire their knowledge, and to assume that we know better than an expert is an act of foolish hubris that could have serious consequences, even deadly ones. But which expert should you trust?

The knowledge of experts is passed on to us through their testimonies, in written (articles and books) or oral (lectures and speeches) forms, but the layperson is not in a position to evaluate the validity of these testimonies. This means that the relationship between the expert and the ordinary citizen is fundamentally one of trust. Very often when we say 'I know X' what I really mean is that 'I trust Y who knows X', even though trust has a different epistemic status than knowledge.

According to the standard 'tripartite' (three-part) definition of knowledge, which goes back to Plato, I can say that I know something to be true, for example the statement 'there has never been a woman president in the USA', if 1) I believe the statement to be true, 2) the statement is in fact true, and 3) I am justified in believing the statement to be true.[2] There are, of course, potential issues with all three parts of the definition, since beliefs, truth, and justifications are contested concepts open to multiple theories and interpretations; but leaving that aside, the key issue is that the conditions for trusting someone are less demanding than knowledge, in the sense that it is easier (and more convenient) to trust someone than to acquire knowledge about something. When it comes to experts, we have no choice but to rely on trust rather than knowledge.

There is some truth in what philosopher John Hardwig says, that when a layperson relies on an expert, that reliance is necessarily 'blind', by which he means that a layperson cannot be rationally justified in trusting an expert.[3] Perhaps Hardwig was being deliberately provocative when he wrote this, and his claim is perhaps too strong, since 'blind' seems very extreme, almost like flipping a coin. Nevertheless this raises an important question: we trust experts because they are experts and we are not, but what is our trust in the experts based on?

We should start by defining what an 'expert' is. Having superior or more extensive knowledge is certainly part of it, but there is more: an expert is someone who also knows what to do with that knowledge, and crucially knows how to apply that knowledge to new questions and problems. The interesting question is what makes a non-expert (a layperson or novice) trust an expert, and *when* should we trust experts? What is that trust based on?

This is a key question in the field of social epistemology. As explained by Alvin Goldman, who among philosophers is considered one of the best experts on the question of experts, there are at least five different sources of evidence that might convince a novice to trust an expert.

1. A novice might be more convinced by the arguments presented by one expert rather than another expert.
2. A novice might be persuaded after hearing the views of other experts on the subject in question.
3. A novice might be impressed by the appraisals of 'meta-experts' of the experts' expertise (including formal credentials such as university degrees, publications, etc.).
4. A novice might take into account the experts' interests and biases vis-à-vis the question at issue.

For example, we tend not to trust those who have a blatant conflict of interests.

5. A novice will take into consideration the experts' previous track records.[4]

Consider the following scenario. I have inherited some money and now I have to decide how to invest it, but I know very little about the world of finance. I'll talk to a number of financial advisors to see which one I find most persuasive. I will then seek the advice of other experts on the recommendations of the financial advisor I found most persuasive. I will then consider the credentials of this financial advisor, explore whether they have any conflict of interests (for example, is she telling me to invest in a company that, by coincidence, she owns and runs), and finally, I will check this financial expert's track record.

All this makes sense, and it highlights a fundamental feature of the novice/expert relationship: the novice's trust of an expert is often based on a second-level trust: to a great extent we trust an expert because other people who we trust tell us that we can trust the expert in question. This is true of culinary recipes, financial or health decision, and crucially even our disposition towards experts during the coronavirus pandemic: we trust public health experts because our government, our GPs, our favourite commentators in the media, our neighbour with a degree in one of the sciences, tell us that we can trust them.

But apart from the obvious issue of infinite regress, we now face two other problems: what happens when experts disagree, and what happens if we don't have much trust in the people who trust the experts?

When experts disagree

Disagreement among experts is more common than we think, even among scientists. Scientists disagree about many things, but usually behind closed doors (for example, at academic conferences) or in specialized publications that are not widely read, so most of us don't get to hear about it. Scientific knowledge is not different from other types of knowledge. It is naive, and even dangerous, to assume that because medical experts have *scientific* knowledge, they have a direct line to the ultimate truth. As Karl Popper once said, science is the *pursuit* of truth, not the dogmatic certainty that we know the truth. Scientific theories are grounded on the best evidence we hold, and we ought to be prepared to change our mind when new evidence comes in. The moment we think we hold the truth, that we have the last word on an issue, we have betrayed the scientific method. And a few centuries before Popper, the same idea was endorsed by the Enlightenment philosopher Voltaire: 'Cherish those who seek the truth but beware of those who find it.'

We should expect experts to disagree, since different experts rely on different bodies of evidence. The fact that experts disagree is not necessarily a bad thing; in fact it should be welcomed. After all, as John Stuart Mill reminded us in *On Liberty*, the last thing we want is to be dogmatic about the truth: without diversity of opinion, 'the meaning of the doctrine itself will be in danger of being lost, or enfeebled, and deprived of its vital effect ... the dogma becoming a mere formal profession, inefficacious for good'.[5] It's a good thing for our views to be challenged, even if one happens to be an expert.

Also, the fact that experts disagree doesn't mean that knowledge can be reduced to subjective opinions. This popular tendency towards effortless relativism, which finds support in Thomas Kuhn's theory of paradigm shifts in the philosophy of science, is not helpful here; in fact – as we shall see – it plays into the hands of populists and their ceaseless attack on elitism.[6] Disagreements among experts occasionally come out into the open, and when that happens the scientific method will eventually adjudicate who was right and who was wrong.

Consider the famous case of Andrew Wakefield, fellow of the Royal College of Surgeons from 1985 and part of a team of researchers in the late 1980s at the University of Toronto. His background and qualifications suggest that he had the trust of other experts in the medical field. In 1998 Wakefield published a paper in the prestigious medical journal *The Lancet* that described eight children whose first symptoms of autism appeared within one month of receiving an MMR (measles, mumps, and rubella) vaccine. From these observations, Wakefield postulated that the MMR vaccine indirectly caused the autism – what he said is that MMR caused intestinal inflammation that led to the translocation of usually non-permeable peptides into the bloodstream and, subsequently, to the brain, where they affected development. Today, after much research, scientists are convinced that there is no link between the MMR vaccine and Autism Spectrum Disorder in children. Wakefield refused to revise his view, and rejected the overwhelming evidence against his initial hypothesis. He was struck off the UK medical register in 2010, and his work on vaccines and autism has been described as an elaborate fraud.[7] But that's not the end of his story. Perhaps not surprisingly he has found an ally in President Trump in the United States, who has strong sympathies with anti-vaccine campaigners: Trump is on the record as saying that 'autism has become an epidemic' and he met with Wakefield during his presidential campaign.[8]

The important point here is that the initial hypothesis linking the MMR vaccine to Autism Spectrum Disorder came from an expert, and that this hypothesis was subsequently contradicted by other experts. On this question, most of us non-experts have no choice but to put our trust in some experts.

In terms of the coronavirus pandemic, experts agree on many things, like the necessity for everyone to wash their hands and the imperative of keeping physical distancing. But they also disagree on other things.[9]

These disagreements are to be expected during this crisis, since coming to a reliable scientific consensus takes time, and there hasn't been enough time for such a consensus to emerge. Consider the mixed messages we are getting from experts on testing or social distancing. Some experts believe that saliva-based tests are the way forward, while others maintain that there is no alternative to the invasive nasopharyngeal (nose and back of the throat) swab test. Regarding distancing, people in France are told that 1 metre social distancing is sufficient, but in Germany 1.5 metres is recommended, and it is 2 metres in Ireland. In some universities, professors are told they should keep 2 metres away from their students, but in lecture theatres it is sufficient for students to keep only 1 metre away from each another.[10] This is scientifically very confusing.

Disagreement between experts creates an epistemic vacuum, which people can take advantage of for their own convenience or personal gain. Let's assume that someone decides that they disagree with the recommendation coming from experts in Ireland, while agreeing with experts in France. Let's assume that experts in Ireland then recommend the wearing of masks in all shops and on public transport. Since this person did not trust the Irish experts on social distancing, they may now be inclined not to trust them on the face mask issue. Other COVID-19 issues where experts disagree include the best time to enforce measures to restrict movement, whether there is significant COVID-19 airborne transmission, or how to flatten the curve of infections rather than merely delaying the peak.

When experts disagree, politicians take centre stage, for better or worse. In Ireland in early October 2020 the National Public Health Emergency Team (Nphet) recommended that the whole country move to Level 5, the highest alert level in the government's strategy with the most stringent restrictions, for four weeks. The government not only rejected this recommendation, raising the alert level from 2 to 3, but speaking on public television Tánaiste Leo Varadkar criticized Nphet, saying its recommendation to move to Level 5 had not been 'thought through'. Time will tell what long-term damage this disparaging remark will inflict on the legitimacy of experts working for Nphet.

The politics of disagreement

'Knowledge is power' is a quote generally attributed to the English philosopher Francis Bacon in 1597.[11] In the previous chapter we saw how some politicians fear truth (hence knowledge), since as Hannah Arendt said, politicians like to maintain the monopoly of power. If knowledge is power, then experts are perceived as a threat, which is why disagreements among experts offer a perfect excuse for politicians to come out from under the shadow of the experts and reclaim the upper hand.

Some politicians are more culpable than others when it comes to distrusting experts. Not surprisingly, populist politicians are more prone to dismiss experts, since experts are part of the 'elite' that populists perceive to be their enemy. In 2016 during the Brexit referendum campaign British politician Michael Gove refused to name any economists who backed Britain's exit from the European Union, saying that 'people in this country have had enough of experts'.[12] Shocking as it sounds, Gove had the last laugh and Brexit was chosen, experts notwithstanding.

Politicians take advantage of disagreements among scientific experts in two ways. First, they use the experts' disagreement to discredit scientific knowledge, with the ultimate aim of replacing science with demagoguery. This is part of the post-truth strategy embraced by Trump and many other populist politicians, as indicated in the previous chapter. Consider the case of climate change. Although there is overwhelming evidence and agreement among experts that climate change is happening, there are still those who reject the evidence, or are paid to reject it. As with anti-vaccine campaigners, there will always be someone in the scientific community prepared to contradict the received view, and politicians will seek them out – rent-an-expert is not as easy as rent-a-crowd, but it can be done.

Secondly, and more importantly for us in terms of the pandemic, when experts disagree a window opens for politicians to choose the experts who best fit their views. This complicates the relationship between experts and novices, since the experts' opinions are filtered by politicians. Even though our trust in politicians is not the same as our trust in scientists, we often have no choice but to go through the politicians before we get to the experts. This would not be the first time that politicians distorted the advice they get from experts for political gain or convenience. Also, we should not assume that scientists are immune from political pressure: not only are scientists affected by general politics, but they are also affected by the internal politics of scientific life.

The situation becomes even more complex because we have multiple disagreements between different types of experts. One does not need to be a scientist to be an expert. Politicians are, in their own way, experts as well. Their job is to pursue the common good (whatever that is) by finding a workable compromise between different factions in civil society, all pursuing their individual interests. Politicians have to communicate their vision of the common good while persuading people to endorse it, and all the time resolving inevitable conflicts. This takes a special skill and expertise, which some have more than others. But the expertise of politicians should never be confused with the expertise of scientists and epidemiologists.

In terms of the present pandemic, we have at least three areas of potential disagreement: first, a disagreement between different scientific experts; secondly, a disagreement between scientific experts and politicians; thirdly, a disagreement between politicians. The layperson is caught between a rock and a hard place, or in this case between a scientific expert and a political expert.

In terms of dealing with COVID-19, inevitably public health experts played a crucial role, but politicians were still able to 'choose' their experts. In the US Trump's refusal to commit to the advice of his health experts, on the basis that America 'wasn't built to be shut down', is a stark reminder of the precarious link between ordinary citizens, politicians, and experts. In the UK, the government sought scientific advice in the form of datasets and highly abstract mathematical models, overlooking experts' advice based on actual experience of real-life medical cases of dealing with respiratory viruses. Mathematical models' predictions are very valuable, but they are not infallible; furthermore they can be less precise than one might think, and the data on which mathematical models run can easily be manipulated to give the desired outcome. This gave the government an excuse to pursue a certain kind of policy as opposed to a different policy.[13]

In Sweden, the government went for a different policy compared to the rest of Europe and the rest of the world, with minimal lockdown. The consequences were dire, and Sweden has one of the highest COVID-19 deaths-per-capita rates in Europe, much higher than the other Scandinavian countries. In early June 2020 Sweden had counted 4,542 deaths and 40,803 infections in a population of 10 million, while Denmark (population 5.8 million) has seen 580 deaths, Norway (population 5.3 million) 237 deaths, and Finland (population

5.5 million) 321 deaths. Anders Tegnell, Sweden's state epidemiologist, in charge of the country's response to COVID-19, admitted that because of Sweden's policies too many people died, and he even came close to issuing an apology when he said that 'If we were to encounter the same disease again, knowing exactly what we know about it today, I think we would settle on doing something in between what Sweden did and what the rest of the world has done.'[14]

This is significant: experts in science and medicine can only advise; it is for experts in politics to decide and choose who they listen to. One of the world's authorities on when experts disagree, philosopher Maria Baghramian of University College Dublin, is right to remind us that policy can only be evidence-informed rather than evidence-based: 'Policymakers often have unrealistic expectations of scientific advice but science is only one form of knowledge that must be integrated with local knowledge and indigenous knowledge to formulate policy solutions.'[15]

Our obligations

The value of science and experts has never been more obvious than in the first few months of 2020. Experts deserve our trust, but when experts disagree, as inevitably they will, the picture becomes less clear. Science thrives on disagreement. As Maria Baghramian rightly points out, 'experts do not need to be in agreement to be trustworthy, nor should we lose trust in them when they get things wrong'.[16] Nevertheless, when experts disagree, politicians pounce on the opportunity to take control and fill the space generated by any ambiguity.

If this crisis has taught us anything, it is that we can never wash our hands of our moral responsibilities. Personal responsibility is a recurring theme in this book, and we touched on it in Chapters 5 and 6 in terms of what are known as alethic obligations: our duty to do our best to hold beliefs that are true or very likely to be true. It is far too easy for politicians to hide behind the scientists, since experts can only advise about very specific issues; it is the politicians' job to make policies.[17] Similarly, it is much too convenient for the layperson to hide behind the politicians, and take advantage of any ambiguity in policies. Given the nature of this crisis, everyone has to play their part. Most of us are not epidemiologists and never will be, but we all have a duty to make an effort to understand, to the best of our abilities, the threat that COVID-19 is posing, and what we can do to stop the virus from spreading.

On top of the alethic obligation, there is also another obligation that applies to all of us, namely, a duty not to cause harm to others. We can call this the obligation of non-maleficence. The concept of non-maleficence in ethics has deep historical roots. The Greek philosopher and physician Hippocrates (c. 460–c. 377 BCE) is universally considered to be the father of Western medicine, and is also credited with formulating the earliest ethical code of conduct for the medical profession, the Hippocratic Oath. The received view today is that the core moral imperative of this oath is captured by the principle *primum non nocere* (first, do no harm), although this well-known maxim is in fact not in the Hippocratic Oath. Something similar to it can be found in Hippocrates' *History of Epidemics*, although not in so many words. In this text Hippocrates says that a physician should aim 'to do good, and not to do harm', which does not have the categorical priority that the phrase 'first, do no harm' suggests.

A few centuries later the same idea resurfaces in the philosophical writing of Cicero: in *De Officiis* (*On Duties*), Cicero argues that the first task of justice is to prevent men from causing harm to others: 'Now the first thing that justice requires of us is this; that no one should do any hurt to another, unless by way of reasonable and just retribution for some injury received from him.'[18] In the last 200 years many influential philosophers, working in very different traditions and schools of thought, have also endorsed the concept of non-maleficence, including J. S. Mill, W. D. Ross, H. L. A. Hart, and Karl Popper.

The non-maleficence obligation is a reminder that there is never an excuse for performing actions that unnecessarily put other people's lives at risk, even if those actions are strictly speaking not forbidden. This has never been more true that during the present pandemic crisis. Not doing one's part in this communal effort is morally reprehensible. No doubt politicians made mistakes, and restrictions could have been introduced sooner, which would have saved many lives; but the fact that there were no travel restrictions, and that large group gatherings were not prohibited until it was too late, is no excuse for going to the Cheltenham races, or to concerts, or meeting friends in the pub. That is morally reckless behaviour, which cannot be excused merely because experts or government officials did not prohibit it. A few days after the lockdown restrictions were lifted in the UK, 6,000 people attended two illegal raves in Manchester.[19] Mild discomfort is not a legitimate reason for not wearing face masks in public spaces, and some of the excuses used to justify this selfish behaviour, for example that it isn't 'the American way', are simply ridiculous. To appeal to the notion of individual freedom and rights as justification for not wearing a face mask reflects a spectacular misunderstanding of the meaning and value of these terms. Coronavirus is highly contagious, but so is stupidity, and they are equally deadly.

Conclusion

At the start of this chapter we said that trust plays a key role in the way we acquire knowledge, so much so that the line between knowledge and trust gets blurred. It will be interesting to see what happens after the pandemic, in terms of society's trust in science and experts. As Baroness Onora O'Neill says, people do not generally reject expertise of all sorts – people who have a tooth problem still want an expert dentist rather than a car mechanic when they want to have that problem fixed – but they tend to snipe at other sorts of expertise.[20]

It is to be hoped that the work and research of experts will be fully appreciated, perhaps for the first time in many years, and there will be a rehabilitation of experts and universities as deserving of society's trust and respect, and of course adequate funding. Putting more resources in education is not just an investment, but a lifeline. Education fosters the kinds of skills in the population at large that allow everyone to make reasonable judgements about who to trust and who not to trust.

But there is also a less auspicious scenario, which sees even more people turning against scientists and other experts. The initial praise that experts and researchers received at the start of this crisis quickly turned to resentment when the advice to enforce a strict lockdown became personally and financially unbearable, fuelled by unscrupulous populist politicians wanting to turn the growing animosity against this perceived elite to their own advantage.

The uncertainty regarding how science will fare post COVID-19 raises an interesting question about the best way to organize politics during crisis management. One of the most distinguished living philosophers of law, Joseph Raz, has suggested radical changes to institutional structures that should enable science to guide policy choices:

Perhaps there should be certain domains regarding which some scientific institutions should take the decisions, guided by a loose framework of policies determined by democratic institutions – in a way analogous to the way in some countries the central bank is autonomous in its decisions, subject to a definition of its general goals, determined by democratic institutions.[21]

I would certainly welcome this.

8

Normal People,
normalized violence

A novel is never anything but a philosophy put into
images.
    Albert Camus, review of *Nausea* by Jean-Paul Sartre

On 27 March 2020 *The Guardian* published a poignant
piece by the Italian novelist Francesca Melandri, entitled 'A Letter to the UK from Italy: This is What We
Know about Your Future'. When this was published
Italy had already been in lockdown for a number of
weeks, while the UK and other countries across Europe
were about to start on this unprecedented public health
measure. Melandri's message was both tender and ago-
nizing. She begins her letter as follows: 'I am writing
to you from Italy, which means I am writing from your
future. We are now where you will be in a few days.
The epidemic's charts show us all entwined in a parallel dance.'[1] She goes on to make a number of predictions, all of which proved right. It was indeed a letter
from the future, and the future unfolded as predicted.

    Here I want to highlight two points from this letter.
First, as all sporting and cultural events stopped

almost overnight, people in lockdown looked for creative ways to pass the time and entertain themselves. After all, there is a limit to what one can watch on Netflix. As Melandri accurately predicted: 'You'll find dozens of social networking groups with tutorials on how to spend your free time in fruitful ways. You will join them all, then ignore them completely after a few days.' This chimes with the experience of millions of people during lockdown: many good intentions, not so many results.

The second point is haunting, because it is presented to us in minimalist terms, as if it is so obvious as not to merit any detailed elaboration. Melandri writes: 'Many women will be beaten in their homes.' Melandri follows this up later with another one-liner, which may or may not be related to the previous point about domestic abuse: 'Many children will be conceived.'

We don't know yet whether more children were conceived during lockdown, but we do know that there was a steep rise in incidents of domestic violence. This phenomenon was universal, although it was worse in some countries than others. Since the start of the pandemic, the United Nations has reported that Lebanon and Malaysia have seen the number of calls to domestic violence helplines double, and in China they have trebled.[2] In Ireland reports of domestic violence increased by almost 25 per cent during the first lockdown in March and April 2020. By October there was an 18 per cent year-on-year increase in the number of domestic issues-related calls to the Irish police, the gardaí.[3] In the UK the largest domestic abuse charity, Refuge, reported a 700 per cent increase in calls to its helpline in a single day, and a separate helpline for perpetrators of domestic abuse seeking help to change their behaviour received 25 per cent more calls after the start of the COVID-19 lockdown.[4]

In what follows, the focus will be on one cultural event that captured the imagination of millions of people during the lockdown, especially in the UK and Ireland. As we will see, domestic violence is an important theme in the work in question.

Normal People, normalized violence

'The voice of a generation' is an accolade often abused, and misused, but it may be true of Irish writer Sally Rooney. Originally published in 2018 and winner of the 2018 Costa novel award, in April 2020 her book *Normal People* was broadcast as a widely acclaimed and successful TV adaptation on BBC3, evocatively directed by Lenny Abrahamson and Hettie Macdonald.[5] A great deal has been written about the loss of innocence of the two main characters, Connell and Marianne, in this modern Irish tale. A political reading, based on class analysis, has also received some attention. And then there is the sex. Lots of sex. And like the sex in the novel, since the television adaptation was aired this aspect of the story has incessantly, relentlessly been written about, talked about, debated, scrutinized, lauded, and vilified in equal measure.

Normal People involves all of the above, but it is also about something else that has not received the attention it merits. This is a story about the impact of domestic violence: how it shatters people's lives, how survivors struggle to cope with its aftermath, and how a moment of violence can persist over time, almost perpetually. Being a social taboo that survivors choose to evade, due to the shame attached to it or because they are in denial, domestic violence is often impalpable, almost imperceptible, but nevertheless ubiquitous.

In the book there are only a few passing references to the violent histories of the two young protagonists. Towards the beginning of their relationship, after the incident in the nightclub, Marianne says to Connell: 'My dad used to hit my mum', and when after a long silence Connell asks, 'Did he ever hit you?', she replies, 'Sometimes'. Her brother is still physically and emotionally abusive towards her, but Rooney tells us that their mother 'decided a long time ago that it is acceptable for men to use aggression towards Marianne as a way of expressing themselves'.

The violence Marianne was subjected to has cast a long shadow on her life. The way the story unfolds can be seen as the long-term repercussions of violence once experienced; Marianne's sexually self-destructive urges are her way of coping with the violence. This is most clearly depicted in her relationship with Jamie, who likes to inflict pain on her during sex, and with her next boyfriend Luke, in Sweden, with whom 'she experiences no more ownership over her own body than if it were a piece of litter'. This urge is also present when she is with Connell; for example, when they are still in school we are told that 'she would have lain on the ground and let him walk over her body if he wanted, he knew that'.

For his part, Connell may not have been a victim of physical violence, but he was subjected to psychological violence, which is often more destructive. Marianne agrees, saying that compared to being hit 'the psychological stuff is more demoralising'. We are told that Connell's grandmother 'hates him for being alive', and that he never met his father. Connell's way of dealing with his past is to raise a protective shield around himself, which accounts for his crippling shyness and the fact that he is constantly afraid of his own emotions.

One of the recurring themes in the conversations between Connell and Marianne is that they desperately want to be normal but cannot be, because they carry with them an overwhelming sense of being 'damaged'. When Connell asks Marianne why she didn't tell him about her brother's violent behaviour, she says: 'I don't know. I suppose I didn't want you to think I was damaged or something. I was probably afraid you wouldn't want me anymore.' As Albert Camus once said, 'Nobody realizes that some people expend tremendous energy merely to be normal'; the main characters in Sally Rooney's novel are the embodiment of Camus's insight into the human condition.

Damage and integrity

The language of 'damage' is appropriate. One of the most important works in philosophy on sexual violence is by Susan Brison, a survivor. In her outstanding book *Aftermath: Violence and the Remaking of a Self*, she analyses the impact on her conception of her 'self' of surviving a nearly fatal attempted sexual murder.[6] Brison wants to tell us that the violence she suffered cannot simply be reduced to the physical harm or injury. Instead, the violence she suffered can best be captured in terms of a violation of integrity, in all its different forms.[7] She tries to make sense of her experience by referring to the self being 'undone' by violence, how the violence she suffered 'demolished' or 'shattered' her world: 'When the trauma is of human origin and is intentionally inflicted ... it not only shatters one's fundamental assumptions about the world and one's safety in it, but it also severs the sustaining connection between the self and the rest of humanity.'[8] Brison goes as far as to tell us that violence destroys the self: 'A perfectly good, intact, life was destroyed.' The language she uses is precise and significant: in order for something to be destroyed, it must first exist as intact; hence the violence is a violation of integrity.[9]

We normally think of violence as something that people do. This, perhaps, explains why academic and non-academic works on violence tend to focus overwhelmingly on the 'act' of violence, and consequently on the agent performing the action in question. Even the definition of violence in the Oxford English Dictionary emphasizes the 'force' of the act and the intentionality of the action: 'The exercise of physical force so as to inflict injury on, or cause damage to, persons or property.'

Reading *Normal People*, we are reminded that there is more to violence than the act of the perpetrator. Violence is above all something that is experienced by its victims and survivors. To view violence as an experience profoundly changes the way we think about violence. Above all, an experience is characterized by a temporal indeterminacy. What starts as an act of violence, with a precise starting and end point, evolves into an experience, with much broader and more unclear boundaries. The experience of violence lives on long after the initial act has ceased.

Via Connell and Marianne, Sally Rooney offers us a subtle, sophisticated, phenomenological analysis of violence in modern Irish society. She is telling us that violence is not just immediately destructive, but also affects our being-in-the-world; it undermines our basic capacities for making sense of the world around us.[10] Violence is an attack on the very conditions of being a self and a subject in the world.

The experience of violence is perceived, internalized, but not always fully understood by its survivor. The perception may diminish in vigour over time, but its traces may never fully vanish. Long after the act of violence has ceased, the experience lingers on.[11] This is the nature of violence: it is temporally indeterminate, and the suffering it brings resonates long after the act is over. These are the ripples of violence, which are invisible to standard accounts, but ever-present in the young lives of Connell and Marianne. Sally Rooney has written a classic novel that speaks to the eternal mysteries of adulthood and sex, but the dominating transformative force in this story is the brutality of violence, and our efforts to normalize it.

Conclusion

Of the long hours of binge watching that marked the experience of many people during the endless days of lockdown, the twelve episodes aired on the BBC and RTÉ of Sally Rooney's *Normal People* will probably be the stand-out memory for those lucky enough to have seen it. Some people have even claimed that the television adaptation was better than the novel. I wouldn't go as far as that, but it was a close run, and it made some of us go back to the novel and read it for a second time.

Television is entertainment, and people needed a distraction during the lockdown. But there is much more to *Normal People* than the impossible love between two young people. In Chapter 4, Thomas Hobbes's state of nature was evoked to make sense of the experience of lockdown, and how a crisis will bring out the worst in people. In that context a reference was made to the spike of domestic violence in those weeks when women and children were confined to live with their abusers, with nowhere to run. We don't know what the long-term impact of this violence will be, but it is not a minor issue. Reading Sally Rooney's novel, and watching its adaptation on television during the lockdown due to COVID-19, touched more nerves than many people may be aware of.

9

Justice after COVID-19

But where some saw abstraction others saw the truth.
Albert Camus, *The Plague*

In the concluding chapter of this book, some considerations will be given to what social, political, and
economic changes need to be made, domestically and
globally, after this pandemic crisis is over. The rhetoric
of war, often used to describe our struggle with COVID-
19, suggests that we must start thinking in terms of
jus post bellum: if life resumes as if this COVID-19
episode was only a temporary glitch, and everything
post COVID-19 goes back to being essentially similar
to life *pre* COVID-19, we will have wasted a unique
opportunity to eradicate some of the worst underlying
conditions of social injustice that inflict misery on bil-
lions of people across the globe. This would be not only
regrettable but unforgivable.

Speaking at the International Labour Organization
Global Summit on 8 July 2020, President of Ireland
Michael D. Higgins made the point that the pandemic
has exposed the stark reality of the paradigm in which

our economies have operated for the last four decades: a shrinking of the space of the state, including the under-valuing of frontline workers: 'From this demonstrably failed model of economy we must free ourselves, make a new balance between economy, ecology, society and culture.'[1] President Higgins is right of course, and more heads of state need to find the courage to call a spade a spade, instead of indulging in nostalgic reminiscences about the 'good ol' days' pre COVID-19 of galloping inequalities and relentless exploitation.

There are many lessons we must learn from the COVID-19 crisis, including things that need to be fixed before the next pandemic comes our way. The main lesson is about the fundamental importance of politics; governing is both an art and a science, and it cannot be left in the hands of opportunistic, incompetent charlatans. More specifically, three aspects of modern politics ought to be prioritized and championed: first, the necessity of a well-funded public administration; secondly, the imperative to raise taxes; thirdly, the requirement to introduce radical reforms, including a universal basic income.

On politics

If COVID-19 has taught us anything, it is that politics matters, and that in times of crisis, political skills can make the difference between life and death. Statistics based on the 'official' death count are unreliable, since some countries deceitfully decided not to include deaths outside hospitals, particularly in care homes. A more reliable set of numbers is the excess mortality rate – the difference between deaths from all causes during the pandemic and the historic seasonal average. In terms of excess deaths the UK at the time of writing has had more than 65,000 deaths from COVID-19, more than any other country in Europe, ahead of Italy and Spain.[2] In Ireland Leo Varadkar's government has been praised for its efforts during this crisis, but when one considers that in the period between 17 February and 3 May 2020 Ireland's excess mortality ranked eighth out of eighteen EU countries, four times that of Denmark and nine times that of Norway, it makes one reconsider.[3] Numbers don't lie. On the other hand, New Zealand did comparatively better than most other countries in the world: on 8 June 2020 Jacinda Ardern announced (with a little dance) that there were no active cases of COVID-19 in New Zealand. This means that COVID-19 has been eradicated from New Zealand. Although a handful of cases resurfaced, on 5 October 2020 Ardern declared that New Zealand had succeeded in beating the virus for a second time.[4]

New Zealand is the place everyone wishes to be right now, the only country that has pursued a 'zero-Covid' strategy with great success. By the end of October 2020 it had had only 1,940 cases and 25 deaths caused by COVID-19, and life is as close to what it was pre-pandemic as you are likely to find anywhere in the world. Ardern was rewarded for her political integrity and competence with a landslide victory for the Labour Party: 49.15 per cent of the votes, 64 seats, and a rare outright parliamentary majority. At the opposite end of the spectrum we find the United States, with 10 million cases and 240,000 deaths.

There are many possible explanations for the success of New Zealand and the failure of the UK, the US, Brazil, Mexico, Peru, and Chile, as well as many other countries in dealing with this virus. These countries will point to geography and population density as mitigating circumstances, and undoubtedly these factors played a role. But we must also allow for political know-how as a determining factor.

While the UK and most other countries in the world aimed for a containment strategy, New Zealand committed from the start to an elimination strategy. New Zealand also introduced harsh restrictions at a very early stage to contain the coronavirus, and it closed its borders. These draconian policies were unpopular at first, and required a good dose of political courage, something that other world politicians lacked.

Politics matters, and in extreme circumstances it can make the difference between life and death. A quick thought-experiment will highlight this point. Let's imagine that you are one of the 50 million people diagnosed with COVID-19. The day before the diagnosis, while shopping in an antique shop, you stumble into a strange-looking contraption. You buy it out of curiosity and take it home. After close inspection you realize that you have bought a time machine. Not only that, it has a special feature that allows you to decide to which country to travel when you go back in time. If you had access to this time machine, and you had been diagnosed with COVID-19, and you could go back to 1 January 2020, where would you go? You probably wouldn't go to Wuhan, nor Milan, nor London, but there is a good chance that you would want to go to New Zealand. Some politicians rise to crises, while for others a crisis only reveals their weaknesses.[5]

Those who are in the 18–25 age group are famously sceptical of politics, a fact fully reflected in their low turnout at elections. Last year I was teaching a group of first year politics students at my university in the autumn semester, with a general election in Ireland only a few weeks away on 8 February. I asked my students how many of them had registered to vote, and roughly 50 per cent raised their hands. According to this admittedly not scientifically accurate experiment, therefore, roughly 50 per cent of my politics students were not registered to vote. This makes one wonder: if not even politics students can be bothered to take part in an election, what does it say about the longevity of democratic politics?[6]

Political apathy is often explained, if not justified, by claims that 'all politicians are the same', therefore 'it makes no difference if I vote or not'. This is not only lazy rhetoric, it is also profoundly wrong. If anything good comes out of this pandemic, it will be that people will realize once again that politics is deadly important, and we should all take it very seriously. If nothing else, it is in our own interest to take politics seriously. The extraordinarily high turnout at the 2020 American presidential election gives us reason to be hopeful.

On the state

If politics matters, so does the state. In political theory the state doesn't always get a good reception, perhaps understandably so. The worst atrocities and acts of injustice are almost always carried out at the hands of the state, from genocides to wars. As Zygmunt Bauman points out in one of the most influential books on the subject, the Holocaust would be inconceivable without the unlimited power inherent in the modern state.[7] The abuse of state power is one reason why anarchism is still a strong tradition in political thought, and one that we discard at our peril.

But as suggested in Chapter 4, anarchism has its limitations. During moments of crisis, notwithstanding admirable community-minded actions at the local level by people motivated by a strong sense of solidarity, a strong case can be made for the need to organize politics around the centralized institution of the modern state. Brian Barry, one of the most astute political theorists of the last generation (and my PhD supervisor at the LSE many years ago), was working on a normative theory of the state to go with his theory of social justice as impartiality when he died in 2009.[8] We get a glimpse of his views on the role of the state from a short lecture he gave in 1991, which was published posthumously only in 2011, and what he has to say is still pertinent and valid.[9]

Barry was only too aware of the political reality at the end of the twentieth century, in which state authority 'leaks away' to sub- and supranational institutions, and in which peoples, societies, and cooperative ventures are not necessarily identical. This is what he referred to as 'differential political authority'.[10] Nevertheless, he held that distributive justice is only possible in states; therefore what is required is different authorities deciding on different issues at different levels. As Barry explains, 'Distributive justice, for example, asks for something that binds people together; there is a relation between the degree of identification and the degree of willingness to give, the degree of redistribution.'[11]

The state, and public institutions more generally, is necessary for two reasons: its ability to coordinate efforts and resources, and its ability to motivate people to contribute to the common good. Both are necessary for social justice, and social justice is the difference between a successful and a less-successful response in moments of crisis. Today we find that in most liberal democracies the private sphere has encroached on the public sphere, with disastrous effects on our democracy. Private industry is doing the jobs that were historically done, and should be done, by public institutions. As Chiara Cordelli highlights in her book *The Privatized State*, many governmental functions today, from the management of prisons and welfare offices to warfare and financial regulation, are outsourced to private entities.[12] Even education and healthcare are funded in part through private philanthropy rather than taxation. This level of privatization constitutes a regression to what philosophers call 'a state of nature'. Constitutional limits on privatization should be a priority.

The COVID-19 pandemic is confirmation, if ever it was needed, that the state can be our best friend in a crisis, and that in fact a proper functioning state is our only hope in fighting future crises of this nature. One of the reasons why the so-called Spanish flu of 1918 killed many more people than the COVID-19 pandemic of 2020 is because a hundred years ago the state did not have the resources it has today, and also because a hundred years ago we could not rely on the instruments of the modern state to orchestrate the efforts necessary to minimize the harm caused by such a virus. Without the state there are only spontaneous actions, which are not sufficient on their own to ensure the necessary level of coordination across society. The state is society's chief coordinator.

Consider another thought-experiment: you have to choose between two worlds with COVID-19. One is the world as we know it today, where politics is organized around a central state, with all its many imperfections. The other is just like ours, except that in this parallel universe there is no central state to issue public health warnings, to access and relay the best scientific advice to its citizens on the necessary measures to stop the spread of the virus, to enforce a lockdown if necessary and provide payments to those economically affected by it, to provide the hospitals, the ventilators, the PPE equipment, and all the apparatus necessary to keep people alive. Which world would you choose? I would choose a world with a state.

The best defence we have against a pandemic is to coordinate our actions, and large-scale coordination cannot be spontaneous; it requires a centralized institution to make it happen. Never before have key state institutions such as a nationalized, public health service been more appreciated and needed. The way forward is to have more state, not less. COVID-19 is a confirmation that we need to organize our social and political affairs around the political philosophy of John Rawls, not Robert Nozick, and the economics of John Maynard Keynes, not Friedrich von Hayek. There is nothing more toxic than the neoliberal political tendency that over the last forty years has seen key state functions slowly but ceaselessly being handed over to the private sphere, which is governed by private interests and not the public good.[13] The time has come to stop this trend and reverse it.

As we start the conversation about rebuilding our society post COVID-19, we must not fall into the trap of being nostalgic about how things were before this pandemic; instead we must seize the moment and start rebuilding our society on a different set of foundational values. As the Kantian philosopher Onora O'Neill has recently suggested, what is required is attention to action that requires wider (and often more demanding) coordination between organizations, including governments, and above all action that crosses borders: 'we need to attend not only to restoring flows of goods and services, but to strengthening the social, political and economic structures for securing co-ordination which have proved vulnerable and could fail again, and to building more robust structures'.[14]

In other words, we need more coordination at all levels, including the sub- and supranational, but we cannot do without a state. In our efforts to rethink the state, I would suggest that one useful place to start is a re-evaluation of Marx's theory of the state.[15]

On taxes

As we move away from the aberrations of neoliberalism, and commence the long-overdue process of revamping centralized state institutions, starting from a well-resourced nationalized health service and education system, taxes will have to go up, especially for the top 30 per cent of earners in our society. Social justice is an expensive commodity, and everyone will have to pay for it. Tax increases for the wealthier strata of society are not a punishment, or an act of revenge, but a re-evaluation of the balance between private interests and the common good. Or, to use terminology from the stock market, a 'correction'.

There are two certainties in life: death and taxes. We talked about the philosophy of death in the Introduction, so now we should talk about the philosophy of taxes. A key function of taxation is to affect the distribution of income and wealth. Unfair distribution of income, or dangerously unequal accumulations of wealth, can and ought to be corrected by taxation. Inequality is perhaps the major threat the West is facing today, more so than international terrorism or nuclear threats from rogue despots. Inequality is also one of the reasons why COVID-19 has been so devastating in so many corners of the world. Taxation is one of the most effective tools to reverse this growing social malignancy.

The pivotal role of taxation in the modern polity cannot be overstated, and over the years numerous thinkers have reasoned that the system of taxation is synonymous with the establishment of modern state-hood. According to economist Joseph Schumpeter (1883–1950) the modern capitalist state is first and foremost a tax state, while sociologist Norbert Elias (1897–1990) considered taxation a necessary condition in the slow process of civilization. Philosophical inquiry in the ethics of taxation is almost as old as philosophy itself, with Plato commenting in Book I of the *Republic* that 'When there is an income tax, the just man will pay more and the unjust less on the same amount of income.'[16] Not surprisingly, many moral philosophers today still feel that taxation is a necessary evil. Three reasons in particular stand out: citizenship, solidarity, justice.

One reason why taxation is indispensable is that it defines citizenship. To be a citizen is to be a member of a political community. As such, citizens are endowed with a set of rights, but also duties. To be a citizen is to enjoy the luxury of state protection. The fact that thousands of people every week risk their lives in the waters of the Mediterranean in search of this elusive good is a constant reminder of the value of citizenship. But this protection comes at a cost, and taxation is what makes it possible for us to enjoy protection and prosper in our community.

Another reason in favour of taxation is that it enhances a spirit of solidarity. By virtue of making a contribution towards the common good all those who pay taxes in a community develop a common bond, cementing trust built upon the principle of reciprocity. This is what Brian Barry was referring to when he said that distributive justice asks for something that binds people together. Taxation, like giving blood, fosters a sense of camaraderie, which in turn defines our social identity and delineates our place in society.

But there is one more reason why taxation is a good idea, strictly on moral grounds: social justice.[17] A key function of taxation is to affect the distribution of income and wealth. As Samuel Scheffler points out, extreme economic inequality is pernicious: 'It threatens to transform us from a democracy into a plutocracy, and it makes a mockery of the ideal of equal citizenship.'[18] Taxation is one of the most effective tools to reverse this growing social malignancy. Some things are simply too important to be left in the hands of the market and private entrepreneurs.[19]

On radical reforms

Finally, we must have the courage to be brave about the way we want to reshape the world. COVID-19 is a warning bell: unless we make radical changes to our economy, things will be much worse next time we have a pandemic, and experts are telling us that it's going to be a question of 'when', not 'if'. Taxation is an important instrument for implementing social justice, but it doesn't go far enough. As political philosopher Martin O'Neill rightly points out, there is much to be done outside the tax system: what is needed are deep structural reforms to disperse economic and political power.[20] One way to do this is through an unconditional basic income given to all citizens of the state.

Spain deserves to be praised because its socialist-led coalition government introduced a form of basic income for the most needy during the extreme lockdown it was forced to impose. Under this policy, at first about 100,000 homes received a monthly payment, ranging between €462 and €1,000, depending on the number of children in the family. In a second phase this was extended to about one million homes, accounting for about 2.3 million people.[21]

While this was a brave and opportune measure, it is inaccurate to call this policy a 'basic income'. The theory of basic income is the brainchild of Belgian philosopher Philippe van Parjis, and the way he conceived it is that basic income, to work properly, must be both universal and unconditional. This means that basic income would be a replacement for the means-tested social welfare system, hence avoiding the stigma of receiving charity from the state.[22] This was not the case in Spain. Nevertheless, the effort to provide a safety net, whereby every person has a guaranteed minimum income, is a step in the right direction. But basic income need not only be an extreme measure wheeled out during desperate times; we need to rethink the basic axioms of our economy, starting from the premise that there are simply not enough jobs to go around, and that those who are lucky enough to have a job will have to contribute through higher taxes so that everyone has a chance to live with dignity and have real opportunities.

Three experts on basic income, Jamie Cooke, Jurgen De Wispelaere, and Ian Orton, offer a convincing argument why there is a unique window of opportunity to introduce basic income, due to the coexistence of three conditions that have never occurred simultaneously in recent social history.[23] First, COVID-19 impacts the whole population (albeit in decidedly unequal ways) and not merely an easily identifiable segment or group. Secondly, the frequent practice of blaming the victim (the poor, the unemployed, the sick, and the disabled, and of course the immigrant) for their dire circumstances is rendered moot when the root cause is a major external shock, in this case a pandemic. Thirdly, COVID-19 has caused an almost global U-turn on the dominant imperative of budget balancing and appears to have sent the austerity paradigm that has governed social spending in the past decade into oblivion. They are right: basic income could be one of the best things to come out of this global tragedy.

Another policy that must be considered in the post COVID-19 world is what is known as community wealth building. The basic idea is to shift the emphasis from redistribution to predistribution: with redistribution great inequalities are allowed to be generated in the capitalist economy, and then the state intervenes to claw back some of these inequalities through taxes; the idea of predestribution is to engineer markets to create fairer outcomes from the beginning.[24] Similarly, the idea of community wealth building is to redesign core institutional relationships in the economy, especially at the local level, in order to produce more egalitarian outcomes as part of the economy's routine operations. The key to community wealth building is to introduce democratic collective ownership of the local economy, including worker cooperatives, community land trusts, and public and community banking.[25]

Universal basic income and community wealth building are only two radical suggestions for rebuilding society on a more equal footing. COVID-19 has exposed the injustice of our current society, and the deadly reality of gross inequalities.[26] In the last analysis, the best vaccine against COVID-19 and future pandemics is less inequality and more social justice.

Epilogue:
A year of COVID-19

I started writing this book at the beginning of the first lockdown, at the end of March 2020. This was partly motivated by a selfish impetus: I wanted to make sense of what was happening around me, and nothing focuses the mind like the process of writing. But there was something else as well; I believed, and still believe, that philosophy has something important to contribute to the ongoing debate on COVID-19. I have written this book in an effort to convince readers that philosophy and philosophers should not be left out of the dream team of experts on this era-defining global crisis. Philosophy has something to say about COVID-19.

My decision to write about a topic no one had written about before, in the midst of the action, in a rapidly changing environment, was decidedly against the recommendations of the German philosopher Georg Wilhelm Friedrich Hegel (1770–1831), who famously said that philosophy is like the owl of Minerva, who 'spreads its wings only with the falling of the dusk'. Minerva is the Roman name for the Greek Athena, goddess of wisdom and philosophy. What Hegel meant is that human beings can come to understand the unfolding of history, through philosophy, only at the end of human history. In other words, and even more bluntly, Hegel was telling us that wisdom comes from hindsight, after events have occurred and mistakes have been made. For Hegel, philosophy comes after the tragedy, to sweep up the mess.[1]

I disagree; my view of philosophy is fundamentally different from Hegel's. It is precisely *during* times of crisis, when we are desperately trying to make sense of things and we are desperately in need of guidance, that we need philosophy most. In fact, that's when philosophy is most useful, and comes into its own. The spirit in which this book was written owes a great deal to the mindset of contemporary philosopher Martha Nussbaum: 'It seems to me that good philosophy will always have a place in the investigation of any matter of deep human importance, because of its commitment to clarity, to carefully drawn distinctions, to calm argument rather than prejudice and dogmatic assertion.'[2]

It is not merely the fact that, as Socrates said, the unexamined life is not worth living. That is true of course, but there is more to philosophy than quenching intellectual curiosity. Philosophical reflection is not something we do only and exclusively for ourselves, for the sake of understanding. Philosophy is also action-guiding; philosophy is praxis.[3]

I like to think of philosophy as the art and science of puzzle solving, where solving the puzzle is not an end in itself, but the first step to action and engagement

with the social world. The core of philosophy is prac-
tical reason. Bertrand Russell was right when he said
that 'to teach how to live without certainty, and yet
without being paralysed by hesitation, is perhaps the
chief thing that philosophy, in our age, can do for those
who study it'.[4] Even though there are no guarantees
of firm answers, philosophy always holds aspirations
towards applicability. The ultimate end of philosophy
is to change the world.

I'm writing this epilogue at the start of the second
lockdown, in November 2020, triggered by an even more
devastating second wave of coronavirus. According
to the website Worldometer, 1.2 million people have
died to date of COVID-19, and more will die in the
months to come. Never before has so much research
been done so quickly on a single topic, by experts in
every country in the world, and yet many questions
about coronavirus and COVID-19 still remain unan-
swered. How did SARS-CoV-2 enter the human population? How can we explain the extreme geographical
variation in COVID-19 mortality rates? What is the
full spectrum of health consequences of COVID-19
infection?[5] These are very important questions, but in
the last few pages of this book I want to focus on two
different questions, which are more philosophically
pertinent. First, is this the time to embrace Stoicism?
Secondly, do we have a moral duty not to become ill?

In 2020 there has been a revival of interest in the
philosophy of Stoicism, and for good reasons. Stoicism
is perfect for a pandemic. As Joe Humphreys points

out, Stoicism is primarily about throwing off the chains of irrational thought.[6] The Stoics are constantly reminding us of two things: one, how lucky we are to be alive, and two, to wish the best for others. For Stoicism, there is a direct correlation between success, or happiness, and becoming more virtuous. As Seneca says: 'wherever there is a human being, there is the opportunity for an act of kindness'.

In times of crisis, we need to be kind to ourselves and to others. That alone should be enough to make us want to find out more about Stoicism, especially now that we are learning to deal with the added pressures and challenges posed by COVID-19. But there is more. 'Keep Calm and Wash Your Hands': this simple mantra captures the year 2020, sensible advice informed by a good dose of old-fashioned stoicism.

Stoicism starts from a simple truth: there are things that are within our control, and things that are not within our control. Stoics are only interested in matters that are under our control. The idea of being in control is very important for the Stoics, since control demands freedom from passion, in other words, reason above emotions. The Greeks had a name for this, *apatheia*: equanimity in the face of what the natural world throws at us. As for things we cannot control, Stoicism teaches us that we must be prepared to accept these events as the will of providence. Once again, the Greeks had a word for this, *ataraxia*: imperturbability, literally 'without trouble' or 'tranquillity'.

With COVID-19 the natural world has thrown a
lethal curve ball at us. Stoicism tells us that we should
keep calm and not let our passions run wild (no panic
buying in supermarkets and no hoarding); that we
should approach the issue rationally (listening to the
experts); that we have a moral duty to do everything
we can to keep ourselves and others safe (washing our
hands and foregoing unnecessary trips abroad). This is
all very sensible, but unfortunately it can also easily be
misunderstood and misapplied.

Learning to accept what is not in our control has
nothing to do with welcoming austerity or self-
denial, as many wrongly assume. Stoicism is not
about embracing dour asceticism, and it is certainly
not the philosophy of withdrawal and inaction. While
Stoicism tells us that we should ultimately accept our
fate, we do so only after putting up a brave fight. The
UK government's bizarre, fatalistic (and no doubt fatal)
policy of 'herd immunity' should never be confused
with Stoicism. This is the philosophical tradition of
Zeno of Citium and Marcus Aurelius, of Cicero and
Seneca, not of Doris Day's 'Che Sera Sera'.

Now to our second question: do we have a moral duty
not to become ill? To answer this question, we must
first explore dominant trends in moral philosophy.
There are two main rival models of ethics: one based
on rights, the other on duties. The rights-based model,
which traces its philosophical origins to the work of
John Locke in the seventeenth century, starts from the
assumption that individuals have rights, specifically

a natural right to 'life, liberty, and property'.[7] This wording influenced Thomas Jefferson in the USA when he drafted the Declaration of Independence in 1776: the first article refers to the unalienable right to 'Life, Liberty and the pursuit of Happiness'.[8] Thanks to Locke and Jefferson, the rights-based approach is still going strong today. In its most zealous libertarian expression it also adds that there are things no person or group (especially the state) may do to individuals without violating their rights.[9]

Putting rights at the centre of morality is attractive, but it can have disconcerting implications. According to the claim-rights approach, duties are correlated to rights, but only in a subordinate role: my right to free speech puts you under a duty to allow me to publish my satirical cartoons; my right to an education puts others under a duty not to throw acid in my face on my way to school; my right to health implies a duty on my country to provide some healthcare services, to the best of my country's abilities. The idea of claim-rights, as defined by the American legal theorist Wesley Hohfeld (1879–1918), is arguably the dominant interpretation in the discourse of rights, including human rights. What is distinctive about the claim-right is that a duty-bearer's duty is 'directed at' or 'owed to' the right-holder.[10]

Rights play a crucial role in modern politics and ethics, and rightly so. We cannot think of modern life in the West without reflecting on hard-won negative and positive rights, including the right to make mistakes. A new law was approved in France in 2018 which gives citizens the 'right to make mistakes' in dealings with the government without being automatically punished. This is to be welcomed.

But what started as a right to life, liberty, property, and the pursuit of happiness has evolved to justify many other claims, including the right to become ill, or at the very least the right to risk getting ill. In the age of COVID-19, this right has been taken to menacing excesses by anti-mask movements, politically active in almost every country around the world. This is the ugly side to rights-based theories. Your right to become ill, or to risk becoming ill, could imply a duty on others to look after you during your illness. In the exceptional times we find ourselves in today, putting rights before duties is beyond the realm of justification. The right to become ill is potentially deadly, and not only for the sick person: in the UK more than 620 NHS staff and social care worker deaths have been linked to coronavirus; in Italy 181 doctors have died from COVID-19; and in the US 1,293 healthcare workers have died from COVID-19. Contrary to what the rights-based model is suggesting, from a moral point of view it is a mistake to think of duties merely as correlated and subordinate to rights.

COVID-19 is forcing us to revisit some of our most entrenched moral assumptions, and embrace new perspectives. The pre-eminence of rights in our moral compass has created an entitlement culture, even vindicating unacceptable levels of selfishness. In a world where people must learn to live with COVID-19, it is imperative to undertake a fundamental duty not to become ill, and do everything in our means to save others from getting ill. Morally speaking, duties should come first and not be subordinated to rights.

The moral senselessness of the anti-mask movement becomes evident in comparison to another crucial right: the right to have sex. We certainly have a right to have sex, but this is not an absolute right. Our right to have sex, assuming that all those involved are competent to give their valid consent, is trumped by a duty not to have sex if you know that you are carrying a sexually transmitted disease, unless you fully disclose this information prior to the sexual act. Similarly, with COVID-19 our right to become ill is trumped by a duty not to put other people's lives at risk, especially those who may be under a duty to look after us.

We are now facing the second wave of the coronavirus, and the second major lockdown. There may be more waves and more lockdowns in the future. As lockdown fatigue sets in, we all need to find strength to keep going. As a philosopher, when the going gets tough I find inspiration in philosophy. Putting duties before rights is not a new, revolutionary idea.[11] On the contrary, it is one of the oldest rules in the book of ethics. As I argued in Chapter 7, the moral principle *primum non nocere*, first do no harm, is the core principle in the Hippocratic Oath, widely attributed to the Greek philosopher and physician Hippocrates.[12] It is also a fundamental principle in the moral philosophy of Marcus Tullus Cicero, who in *De Officiis* argues that the first task of justice is to prevent men from causing harm to others. When it comes to navigating the morality of living with COVID-19, we could do a lot worst than take a leaf out of the moral teachings of our philosophical ancestors.

Notes

Notes to Chapter 1

1 The Latin quote is 'disiungamusque nos a corporibus, id est consuescamus mori' (*Tusculan Disputations*, Book I, 31), which is sometimes translated literally as 'to separate the soul from the body is the same thing as learning how to die'; see Cicero, *On Living and Dying Well*, Penguin, 2012, p. 37. However, the more popular translation is the one I give in the text.

2 The statistics on coronavirus throughout this book are taken from this website: https://www.worldometers.info/coronavirus/.

3 On Cicero's life, see Anthony Everitt, *Cicero: The Life and Times of Rome's Greatest Politician*, Random House, 2003. On Tullia and Cicero's relationship with his daughter, see Susan Treggiari, *Terentia, Tullia and Publilia: The Women of Cicero's Family*, Routledge, 2007.

4 On Montaigne and humanism, see John O'Brien, 'The humanist tradition and Montaigne', in *The Oxford Handbook of Montaigne*, ed. Philippe Desan, Oxford University Press, 2016.

5 This quote is from Michel de Montaigne, *The Complete Essays*, Penguin, 1993, p. 96.

6 Ibid., p. 96.

7 On philosophical explorations of death, see Shelly Kagan, *Death*, Yale University Press, 2012. For a series of lectures by Professor Kagan on death, see https://campuspress.yale.edu/shellykagan/death/.

Notes

NOTES TO CHAPTER 2

1 In his book *Poverty and Famines: An Essay on Entitlement and Deprivation*, Oxford University Press, 1981, Amartya Sen argues that famines are not caused by scarcity of food supply, but by political factors. Democracies do not always solve all the problems of hunger and malnutrition, but famines are less likely to occur in democracies.

2 Judith Shklar, *The Faces of Injustice*, Yale University Press, 1990.

3 Ibid., p. 4.

4 'Justice is the first virtue of social institutions, as truth is of systems of thought. A theory however elegant and economical must be rejected or revised if it is untrue; likewise laws and institutions no matter how efficient and well-arranged must be reformed or abolished if they are unjust.' John Rawls, *A Theory of Justice*, Harvard University Press, 1971, p. 3.

5 'We overlook the reach and the complexity of injustice, we impoverish our understanding of it, when we instinctively obey the arbitrary dictates of etymology, theorising injustice as a sheer negation of something else.' E. Heinz, *The Concept of Injustice*, Routledge, 2013, p. 6.

6 This reversal of roles has the approval of another influential political philosopher, Nancy Fraser: 'we do experience injustice, and it is only through this that we form an idea of justice ... Only when we contemplate what it would take to overcome injustice does our otherwise abstract concept of justice acquire any content.' 'On justice', *New Left Review*, 74, March–April 2012, p. 43.

7 Vittorio Bufacchi, *Social Injustice*, Palgrave, 2012.

8 Iris Marion Young, *Justice and the Politics of Difference*, Princeton University Press, 1990.

9 On Black Lives Matter, see Alexander Blanchard, 'Black Lives Matter and the politics of violence', *New Statesman*, 17 June 2020, https://www.newstatesman.com/international/politics/2020/06/black-lives-matter-politics-violence-police-structural-racism.

10 Here I'm paraphrasing Brian Barry, who makes a similar point about social justice. As he says: 'We cannot separate the question "What is justice?" from the question "Why be just?"' *Theories of Justice*, University of California Press, 1989, p. 358.

11 I discuss this three-dimensional framework of social injustice in chapter 1 of my book *Social Injustice*.

12 On the injustice of industrial schools and Magdalene laundries in Ireland, see www.jfmresearch.com. See also Patsy McGarry, 'Magdalene laundries: "I often wondered why were they so cruel"', *The Irish Times*, 6 June 2018, https://www.irishtimes.com/news/social-affairs/religion-and-beliefs/magdalene-laundries-i-often-wondered-why-were-they-so-cruel-1.3521600.

13 For a critique of meritocracy, see Brian Barry, *Why Social Justice Matters*, Polity, 2005, ch. 10, 'Responsibility vs. equality?'

14 On the lack of access to clean water, see https://www.who.int/news-room/detail/18-06-2019-1-in-3-people-globally-do-not-have-access-to-safe-drinking-water-unicef-who.

15 Mike Davis, *Planet of Slums*, Verso, 2017, p. 13.

16 Friedrich Engels, *The Condition of the Working Class in England*, Penguin, 2009, p. 184.

17 Ibid., p. 143.

18 Ibid.

19 Quoted in Octávio Luiz Motta Ferraz, 'Pandemic inequality: the two worlds of social distancing', *The Yale Review*, 3 April 2020, https://yalereview.yale.edu/pandemic-inequality.

20 On Kenya and COVID-19, see Nita Bhalla, 'Futures destroyed: COVID-19 unleashes "shadow pandemics" on Africa's girls', Thomson Reuters Foundation News, 20 August 2020, https://news.trust.org/item/20200820135640-yl2ii/; Nita Bhalla, 'Kenya orders probe into rise in violence against women and girls during pandemic', Reuters, 6 July 2020, https://www.reuters.com/article/us-health-coronavirus-kenya-women-trfn-id USKBN2472ER; Neha Wadekar, 'Kenya is trying to end child marriage. But climate change is putting more young girls at risk', *Time*, 12 August 2020, https://time.com/5878719/climate-change-kenya-child-marriage/.

21 The World Bank has so far loaned money to about a hundred countries, accounting for 70 per cent of the world's population, but that may not be enough.

22 On how women's voices have been marginalized in COVID-19 media coverage, see https://www.opendemocracy.net/en/5050/womens-voices-marginalised-in-media-reporting-of-coronavirus/.

23 Miranda Fricker, *Epistemic Injustice: Power and the Ethics of Knowing*, Oxford University Press, 2007.

24 On the class divide in the COVID-19 death rate, see Mark Williams, 'Coronavirus class divide – the jobs most at risk of contracting and dying from COVID-19', *The Conversation*, 19 May 2020, https://theconversation.com/coronavirus-class-divide-the-jobs-most-at-risk-of-contracting-and-dying-from-covid-19-138857.

25 On the possible link between ethnic minorities, air pollution and COVID-19 in the UK, see Damian Carrington, 'Covid-19 impact on ethnic minorities linked to housing and air pollution', *The Guardian*, 19 July 2020, https://www.theguardian.com/world/2020/jul/19/covid-19-impact-on-ethnic-minorities-linked-to-housing-and-air-pollution.

26 On COVID-19 and disability, see https://www.disabilitynewsservice.com/coronavirus-academics-call-for-urgent-inquiry-into-deaths/.

27 On the divide in the COVID-19 death rate in the US between black Americans and the rest of the nation, see Ed Pilkington, 'Black Americans dying of Covid-19 at three times the rate of white people', *The Guardian*, 20 May 2020, https://www.theguardian.com/world/2020/may/20/black-americans-death-rate-covid-19-coronavirus.

28 On how COVID-19 is putting food delivery riders at serious health risk, see Caterina Morbiato, 'Delivering food in a pandemic', *Jacobin*, 9 May 2020, https://jacobinmag.com/2020/05/food-delivery-workers-italy-bologna-coronavirus.

29 On inadequate ventilators in the UK, see Peter Foster and Michael Pooler, 'Ventilator standards set out for UK makers "of no use" to Covid patients', *Financial Times*, 15 April 2020, https://www.ft.com/content/365529f8-bff3-41d2-949f-d0eedff0cfbb.

30 On inadequate PPE from Turkey, see Kevin Rawlinson, 'Coronavirus PPE: all 400,000 gowns flown from Turkey for NHS fail UK standards', *The Guardian*, 7 May 2020, https://www.theguardian.com/world/2020/may/07/all-4000 00-gowns-flown-from-turkey-for-nhs-fail-uk-standards.

31 On the inadequate preparedness for this pandemic, see this interview with Carlo Caduff, medical anthropologist and associate professor at King's College London, https:// allegralaboratory.net/on-pandemic-prophecy-unsustainable- lockdowns-and-the-magic-of-numbers-a-conversation-with- carlo-caduff/; on privatization and inadequate preparedness for this pandemic, see Felicity Lawrence et al., 'How a decade of privatisation and cuts exposed England to coronavirus', *The Guardian*, 31 May 2020, https://www.theguardian.com/ world/2020/may/31/how-a-decade-of-privatisation-and-cuts- exposed-england-to-coronavirus.

32 Oxfam on richest top 1 per cent: https://www.oxfam.org/en/ press-releases/richest-1-percent-bagged-82-percent-wealth- created-last-year-poorest-half-humanity.

33 Top 1 per cent in the US: https://www.bloomberg.com/ news/articles/2019–11–09/one-percenters-close-to-surpass ing-wealth-of-u-s-middle-class.

34 Top 1 per cent in the UK: Larry Elliott, 'Top 1% of earners in UK account for more than a third of income tax', *The Guardian*, 13 November 2019, https://www.theguardian. com/business/2019/nov/13/richest-britain-income-tax-reve nues-institute-fiscal-studies.

35 On UK billionaires financing the Conservative Party, see Rob Merrick, 'Conservatives branded "party of billionaires" as one-third of UK's richest people donate to Tories', *The Independent*, 19 November 2019, https://www.independent. co.uk/news/uk/politics/conservatives-general-election-dono rs-billionaire-john-mcdonnell-labour-a9208036.html.

36 UK worst hit by COVID-19: John Burn-Murdoch and Chris Giles, 'UK suffers second-highest death rate from coronavi- rus', *Financial Times*, 28 May 2020, https://www.ft.com/ content/6b4c784e-c259-4ca4-9a82-648ffde71bfo.

37 On Stoicism in a time of pandemic, see Joe Humphreys, 'Coronavirus: how can philosophy help us in this time of

crisis?', *The Irish Times*, 26 March 2020, https://www.irish times.com/culture/coronavirus-how-can-philosophy-help-us-in-this-time-of-crisis-1.4205889. See also Donald Robertson, 'Stoicism in a time of pandemic: how Marcus Aurelius can help', *The Guardian*, 25 April 2020, https://www.the guardian.com/books/2020/apr/25/stoicism-in-a-time-of-pan demic-coronavirus-marcus-aurelius-the-meditations; and Donald Robertson, 'Stoicism amid pandemic panic', *iainews*, 87, 10 April 2020, https://iai.tv/articles/stoicism-amid-pan demic-panic-auid-1436.

NOTES TO CHAPTER 3

1 The statistics on global population ageing are from https://www.un.org/en/development/desa/population/publications/pdf/ageing/WPA2017_Highlights.pdf.
2 A copy of the guidelines issued by the Italian College of Anaesthesia, Analgesia, Resuscitation and Intensive Care (SIAARTI) can be found at http://www.siaarti.it/SiteAssets/News/COVID19%20-%20documenti%20SIAARTI/SIAAR TI%20-%20Covid19%20-%20Raccomandazioni%20di%20 etica%20clinica.pdf.
3 On age considerations being considered for Covid patients in the US, see https://www.npr.org/2020/03/21/819645036/u-s-hospitals-prepare-guidelines-for-who-gets-care-amid-cor onavirus-surge.
4 On why the criteria adopted by SIAARTI from an ethical point of view were neither unprecedented nor revolutionary, see Silvia Camporesi, 'It didn't have to be this way', *AEON*, https://aeon.co/essays/a-bioethicist-on-the-hidden-costs-of-lockdown-in-italy. See also Chiara Mannelli, 'Whose life to save? Scarce resources allocation in the COVID-19 out-break', *Journal of Medical Ethics*, 46.6, 2020, pp. 364–6. Mannelli argues for the need for medical ethics consultants in healthcare structures to support the evaluations and deci-sions of healthcare professionals, especially prioritization, since the burden of choice can no longer be put on health-care professionals' shoulders.
5 On the controversy regarding herd immunity in the UK,

see Peter Walker, 'No. 10 denies claim Dominic Cummings argued to "let old people die"', *The Guardian*, 22 March 2020, https://www.theguardian.com/politics/2020/mar/22/ no-10-denies-claim-dominic-cummings-argued-to-let-old-people-die.

6 Mike Ryan, on why herd immunity is dangerous, quoted in https://edition.cnn.com/world/live-news/coronavirus-pande mic-05-11-20-intl/h_15f81e322ab9925b18772fc7f10cf926?fbc lid=IwAR0hLewYj-Mcis44JN96iQ1ANPLJsXz9OssHHGMU cEYBqJIU_vRrMO1_X_Y.

7 Richard Coker, '"Harvesting" is a terrible word – but it's what has happened in Britain's care homes', *The Guardian*, 8 May 2020, https://www.theguardian.com/commentisfr ee/2020/may/08/care-home-residents-harvested-left-to-die-uk-government-herd-immunity.

8 On inadequate resources and lack of protective equipment in care homes in the UK, see Patrick Butler, 'English care bosses say lack of resources cost thousands of lives', *The Guardian*, 11 June 2020, https://www.theguardian.com/society/2020/ jun/11/english-care-bosses-say-lack-of-resources-cost-thou sands-of-lives. See also Lucy Pocock, 'Care homes have long been neglected – the pandemic has shown us how bad things are', *The Conversation*, 8 July 2020, https://theconversation. com/care-homes-have-long-been-neglected-the-pandemic-h as-shown-us-how-bad-things-are-1374585.

9 Marcus Tullius Cicero, 'On old age', in *Cicero: Selected Works*, trans. Michael Grant, Penguin, 1971, p. 220.

10 Ibid., p. 226.

11 Ibid., p. 216.

12 Ibid., p. 229.

13 On Fauci and Trump, see Stephen Collinson, 'Trump's rebuke of Fauci encapsulates rejection of science in virus fight', *CNN Politics*, 14 May 2020, https://edition.cnn. com/2020/05/14/politics/donald-trump-anthony-fauci-scie nce-coronavirus/index.html.

14 On Trump calling Fauci an idiot, see Michael Scherer and Josh Dawsey, 'Trump attacks "Fauci and all these idiots," says public is tired of pandemic, public health restrictions as infection rates rise', *Washington Post*, 20 October 2020,

Notes

https://www.washingtonpost.com/politics/trump-fauci-cam
paign-biden/2020/10/19/30b2fe58-1226-11eb-82af-8646520
63d61_story.html.

15 Martha Nussbaum, *The Monarchy of Fear: A Philosopher Looks at Our Political Crisis*, Simon and Schuster, 2018; Bernard Williams, *Truth and Truthfulness*, Princeton University Press, 2001; Onora O'Neill, *Constructing Authorities: Reason, Politics, and Interpretation in Kant's Philosophy*, Cambridge University Press, 2015.

16 Joseph Raz, *The Morality of Freedom*, Oxford University Press, 1980.

17 J. B. Schneewind, *The Invention of Autonomy*, Cambridge University Press, 1998.

18 Judith Butler, *Precarious Life*, Verso, 2004; *Vulnerability in Resistance*, ed. Z. Gambetti and L. Sabsay, Duke University Press, 2016.

19 Eva Kittay, *Love's Labor: Essays on Women, Equality and Dependency*, Routledge, 1999, p. xi.

20 Martha Albertson Fineman, *The Autonomy Myth: A Theory of Dependency*, The New Press, 2004; Adriana Cavarero, *Inclinations: A Critique of Rectitude*, Stanford University Press, 2016.

21 Cicero, 'On old age', p. 238.

Notes to Chapter 4

1 On UN Secretary General António Guterres and the fear that COVID-19 is threatening global peace and security, see https://news.un.org/en/story/2020/04/1061502.

2 On the risk of civil disorder triggered by local lockdowns in the second wave of the virus, see Clifford Stott, 'Local lockdowns could lead to civil disorder', *The Conversation*, 29 June 2020, https://theconversation.com/local-lockdowns-could-lead-to-civil-disorder-heres-why-141305.

3 On the October 2020 Manchester lockdown, see Paul Mason, 'Andy Burnham spoke the language of class struggle – Labour must follow', *New Statesman*, 21 October 2020, https://www.newstatesman.com/politics/devolution/

162

2020/10/andy-burnham-spoke-language-class-struggle-labou
r-must-follow.

4 And even if COVID-19 doesn't bring down civil society, the collapse of civilization is the most likely outcome of climate change, and much sooner than we think; see https://voiceofac tion.org/collapse-of-civilisation-is-the-most-likely-outcome-top-climate-scientists/.

5 Anne Enright, 'Disaster brings out the best in people', *The Guardian*, 13 June 2020, https://www.theguardian.com/ books/2020/jun/13/overcoming-fears-discovering-nature-wh at-i-have-learned-from-lockdown.

6 On the surge of domestic violence during the lockdown, see Amanda Taub, 'A new Covid-19 crisis: domestic abuse rises worldwide', *New York Times*, 6 April 2020, https://www. nytimes.com/2020/04/06/world/coronavirus-domestic-viole nce.html.

7 On Michel de Montaigne and the plague of 1585, see Robert Zaretsky, 'Montaigne fled the plague, and found himself', *New York Times*, 28 June 2020, https://www. nytimes.com/2020/06/28/opinion/montaigne-plague-essays. html.

8 On Hobbes's frontispiece, see Thomas Poole, 'Leviathan in lockdown', *LRB* blog, 1 May 2020, https://www.lrb.co.uk/ blog/2020/may/leviathan-in-lockdown.

9 Thomas Hobbes, *Leviathan*, Hackett, 1994, Book I, ch. 16, par. 13, p. 104.

10 On anarchism and non-violence, see Carl Joachim Friedrich, 'The anarchist controversy over violence', *Zeitschrift für Politik*, 19.3, 1972, pp. 167–77.

11 On anarcho-ecology, see Henry David Thoreau, *Walden*, Penguin, 2016. See also Arnaud Baubérot, 'The roots of anar chist environmentalism: Louis Rimbault and vegan com munities in France in the first half of the 20th century', *Le Mouvement Social*, 246.1, 2014, pp. 63–74.

12 For a fascinating analysis of case studies of anarchism during the COVID-19 crisis in the United States, see Nathan Jun and Mark Lance, 'Anarchist responses to a pan demic: the COVID-19 crisis as a case study in mutual aid', *Kennedy Institute of Ethics Journal*, special issue on Ethics,

Notes

Pandemics, and COVID-19, forthcoming, https://kiej.george
town.edu/anarchist-responses-COVID-19-special-issue.

13 Hobbes, *Leviathan*, Book I, ch. 13, par. 8, p. 76.

14 On countries aggressively outbidding each other on the
global market for coronavirus protective equipment, see
Kim Willsher et al., 'US accused of "modern piracy" after
diversion of masks meant for Europe', *The Guardian*, 4 April
2020, https://www.theguardian.com/world/2020/apr/03/ma
sk-wars-coronavirus-outbidding-demand.

15 On the US buying up world stock of a key COVID-19 drug,
see Sarah Boseley, 'US secures world stock of key Covid-19
drug remdesivir', *The Guardian*, 30 June 2020, https://www.
theguardian.com/us-news/2020/jun/30/us-buys-up-world-st
ock-of-key-covid-19-drug.

16 On anti-lockdown protests in the United States, see Firmin
DeBrabander, 'The great irony of America's armed anti-
lockdown protesters', *The Atlantic*, 13 May 2020, https://
www.theatlantic.com/ideas/archive/2020/05/guns-proteste
rs/611560/.

17 Hobbes, *Leviathan*, Book I, ch. 13, par. 8, p. 76.

18 On Andrés Manuel López Obrador and COVID-19, see
https://www.worldpoliticsreview.com/articles/28757/for-me
xico-s-amlo-popularity-hinges-on-covid-19-response.

19 Rutger Bregman, *Humankind: A Hopeful History*,
Bloomsbury, 2020.

20 For a comparison of Hobbes and Rousseau on the state of
nature, see Robin Douglass, 'Hobbes vs Rousseau: are we
inherently evil?', *iainews*, 72, 19 March 2019, https://iai.tv/
articles/hobbes-vs-rousseau-are-we-inherently-evil-or-good-
auid-1221.

21 David Hume, *A Treatise of Human Nature*, Clarendon
Press, 1978, p. 495. On Hume's circumstances of justice,
see Brian Barry, *Theories of Justice*, University of California
Press, 1989, ch. 4, 'Hume on justice'.

22 Hobbes, *Leviathan*, Book I, ch. 13, par. 2, p. 75.

23 Max Weber, 'Politics as a vocation' (1918), in H. Gerth
and C. Mills (eds), *From Max Weber: Essays in Sociology*,
Routledge, 2007, pp. 77–128.

24 Hobbes, *Leviathan*, Book I, ch. 13, par. 4, p. 80.

Notes

25 Joe Humphreys, 'COVID-19 shows kindness can be enough to get us through', *The Irish Times*, 30 June 2020, https://www.irishtimes.com/opinion/covid-19-shows-kindness-can-be-enough-to-get-us-through-1.4291682.

Notes to Chapter 5

1 This chapter focuses exclusively on right-wing populism. For a sympathetic analysis of left-wing populism, see Chantal Mouffe, *For a Left-Populism*, Verso, 2018.
2 On populism as an ideology, see Cas Mudde and Cristóbal Rovira Kaltwasser, *Populism: A Very Short Introduction*, Oxford University Press, 2017. See also Daniele Albertazzi and Duncan McDonnell (eds), *Twenty-First Century Populism*, Palgrave, 2007. On the alternative view that populism is not an ideology but a mentality, see Marco Tarchi, 'Populism: ideology, political style, mentality?', *Politologicky Casopis*, 23.2, 2016, pp. 95–109.
3 On 'the pure people' versus 'the corrupt elite', see Cas Mudde, 'The populist zeitgeist', *Government & Opposition*, 39.4, 2004, pp. 541–63.
4 Nadia Urbinati, 'Democracy and populism', *Constellations*, 5.1, 1998, pp. 110–24. See also Nadia Urbinati, *Me the People: How Populism Transforms Democracy*, Harvard University Press, 2019.
5 William Galston, *Anti-Pluralism: The Populist Threat to Liberal Democracy*, Yale University Press, 2018, p. 11.
6 Daniele Archibugi and Marco Cellini, 'How dangerous is populism for democracy?', *Global-e*, 11.21, 10 April 2018, https://www.21global.ucsb.edu/global-e/april-2018/how-dangerous-populism-democracy.
7 Margaret Canovan, 'Trust the people! Populism and the two faces of populism', *Political Studies*, 47, 1999, pp. 2–16. See also Margaret Canovan, *The People*, Polity, 2005.
8 Mary Beard, *SPQR*, Profile, 2016, p. 281.
9 For more on this, see Vittorio Bufacchi, 'Populism and the politically excluded: lessons from Ancient Rome', *Global-e*, 11.29, 29 May 2018, https://www.21global.ucsb.

edu/global-e/may-2018/populism-and-politically-excluded-lessons-ancient-rome.

10 Colleen Shogan, 'Anti-intellectualism in the modern presidency: a Republican populism', *Perspectives on Politics*, 5.2, 2007, pp. 295–303.

11 On Trump's anti-intellectualism, see John L. Campbell, *American Discontent: The Rise of Donald Trump and Decline of the Golden Age*, Oxford University Press, 2018, p. 99.

12 Marc Fisher, 'Donald Trump doesn't read much. Being president probably wouldn't change that', *Washington Post*, 17 July 2016, https://www.washingtonpost.com/politics/donald-trump-doesnt-read-much-being-president-probably-wouldnt-change-that/2016/07/17/d2ddf2bc-4932-11e6-90a8-fb84201e0645_story.html.

13 On Bolsonaro's homophobia, see https://www.bloomberg.com/news/articles/2018-10-27/gays-for-bolsonaro-why-many-will-overlook-his-homophobic-rants.

14 Cas Mudde, 'Will the coronavirus "kill populism"? Don't count on it', *The Guardian*, 27 March 2020, https://www.theguardian.com/commentisfree/2020/mar/27/coronavirus-populism-trump-politics-response.

15 Allan C. Stam, 'Coronavirus and international populism: ideological and generational divides', *Global-e*, 13.32, 26 May 2020, https://www.21global.ucsb.edu/global-e/may-2020/coronavirus-and-international-populism-ideological-and-generational-divides.

16 Paulina Ochoa Espejo, 'Teflon populism: will it slip or falter?', *Global-e*, 13.43, 7 July 2020, https://www.21global.ucsb.edu/global-e/july-2020/teflon-populism-will-it-slip-or-falter.

17 Rogers Brubaker, 'Paradoxes of populism during the pandemic', *Thesis Eleven*, 13 July 2020, https://thesiseleven.com/2020/07/13/paradoxes-of-populism-during-the-pandemic/.

18 Jennifer Finney Boylan, 'Trump and the Boaty McBoatfacing of America', *New York Times*, 28 October 2020, https://www.nytimes.com/2020/10/28/opinion/trump-boaty-mcboatface.html.

19 On the impact of coronavirus in Brazil, and how this may affect

President Bolsorano, see Alfredo Saad Filho, 'Coronavirus: how Brazil became the second worst affected country in the world', *The Conversation*, 29 June 2020, https://thecon versation.com/coronavirus-how-brazil-became-the-second-worst-affected-country-in-the-world-141102.

20 On the idea that we may be witnessing the beginning of the end of Donald Trump, see Franklin Foer, 'The Trump regime is beginning to topple', *The Atlantic*, 6 June 2020, https://www.theatlantic.com/ideas/archive/2020/06/how-re gime-change-happens/612739/.

21 For Tova O'Brien's television interview with Jami-Lee Ross, see https://www.theguardian.com/world/2020/oct/24/tova-obrien-my-feral-interview-with-covid-19-denier-jami-lee-ross.

22 For Danielle Allen's views on how the pandemic will reshape American society, see her interview at https://www. politico.com/news/magazine/2020/07/01/coronavirus-pa ndemic-democracy-america-expert-347431. See also this report she co-authored for the American Academy of Arts and Sciences: https://www.amacad.org/ourcommonpurpose/report.

23 On empirical evidence of the decline in populism in 2020, see Jon Henley and Pamela Duncan, 'European support for populist beliefs falls, YouGov survey suggests', *The Guardian*, 26 October 2020, https://www.theguardian.com/world/2020/oct/26/european-support-for-populist-beliefs-fal ls-yougov-survey-suggests.

24 Gideon Rachman argued in the *Financial Times*, 29 June 2020, that coronavirus could kill off populism; see https://www.ft.com/content/3bcf2b5e-e5f1-48e4-bb15-cd29615a91 98. Rachman quotes Francis Fukuyama who recently said that 'The COVID-19 epidemic may actually lance the boil of populism', and Matthew Goodwin, who believes that 'Liberalism is back. Populism is out.'

Notes to Chapter 6

1 George Orwell, 'Politics and the English language', in *Collected Essays*, Secker & Warburg, 1961 [1946]. Orwell's

essays can be found at https://www.orwell.ru/library/essays/politics/english/e_polit/.

2 On post-sexuality, see P. Maniglier, 'Political and theoretical introduction to post-sexuality', in B. Mousli and E. A. Roustang-Stoller (eds), *Women, Feminism, and Femininity in the 21st Century: American and French Perspectives*, Palgrave, 2009, pp. 201–17.

3 Bill Clinton's White House announcement to the nation can be found at https://www.youtube.com/watch?v=VBe_guezGGc.

4 For a full analysis of this definition of post-truth, see Vittorio Bufacchi, 'Truth, lies and tweets: a consensus theory of post-truth, *Philosophy and Social Criticism*, forthcoming 2020. Online first: https://journals.sagepub.com/doi/full/10.1177/0191453719896382.

5 Hannah Arendt, 'Truth and politics', in *The Portable Hannah Arendt*, ed. Peter Baehr, Penguin, 2000 [1967], pp. 545–75.

6 Ibid., p. 555.

7 On COVID-19 originating in a Chinese lab, see https://www.forbes.com/sites/jackbrewster/2020/05/10/a-timeline-of-the-covid-19-wuhan-lab-origin-theory/#5be476b55aba.

8 On Trump's suggestion of injecting disinfectant into the body, see https://www.bbc.com/news/world-us-canada-52407177.

9 On the survey conducted by the Centers for Disease Control and Prevention (CDC), see https://www.sciencetimes.com/articles/25966/20200606/gargle-bleach-39-surveyed-americans-engaged-risky-cleaning-habits.htm.

10 On Trump and hydroxychloroquine, see https://www.cnbc.com/2020/05/18/trump-says-he-takes-hydroxychloroquine-to-prevent-coronavirus-infection.html. See also https://www.statnews.com/2020/06/05/hydroxychloroquine-had-no-benefit-for-hospitalized-covid-19-patients-possibly-closing-door-to-use-of-drug/.

11 On hydroxychloroquine in Brazil, see Katherine Fung, 'Brazil's Bolsonaro expands use of controversial hydroxychloroquine after daily coronavirus deaths in country hit record high', *Newsweek*, 20 May 2020, https://www.newsweek.

com/brazils-bolsonaro-expands-use-controversial-hydroxyc
hloroquine-after-daily-coronavirus-deaths-1505394.

12 On the risks posed when politics, communication
and entertainment become barely distinguishable, see
Ignas Kalpokas, *A Political Theory of Post-Truth*, Palgrave,
2019.

13 On Facebook spreading fake news, see https://www.forbes.
com/sites/traversmark/2020/03/21/facebook-spreads-fake-
news-faster-than-any-other-social-website-according-to-new-
research/#1ae3890a6e1a.

14 On redefining social networks as 'publishers', see Adrienne
Lafrance, 'The most powerful publishers in the world don't
give a damn', *The Atlantic*, 8 August 2018, https://www.the
atlantic.com/technology/archive/2018/08/the-most-powerf
ul-publishers-in-the-world-dont-give-a-damn/567095/.

15 On alethic obligations, see Maria Paola Ferretti, *The Public
Perspective: Public Justification and the Ethics of Belief*,
Rowman and Littlefield, 2018.

16 On whether facts will make a comeback after the crisis is
under control, see https://www.theglobalist.com/coronavi
rus-pandemic-covid19-media-social-media-misinformation-
post-truth-populism/.

17 Chrysalis L. Wright, 'COVID-19 fake news and its impact on
consumers', *Psychology Today*, 30 April 2020, https://www.
psychologytoday.com/ie/blog/everyday-media/202004/covi
d-19-fake-news-and-its-impact-consumers.

NOTES TO CHAPTER 7

1 On the claim that enforcing the UK's lockdown one week
earlier could have saved 20,000 lives, see Heather Stewart
and Ian Sample, 'Coronavirus: enforcing UK lockdown
one week earlier "could have saved 20,000 lives"', *The
Guardian*, 10 June 2020, https://www.theguardian.com/
world/2020/jun/10/uk-coronavirus-lockdown-20000-lives-
boris-johnson-neil-ferguson.

2 On the standard tripartite definition of knowledge, see
Duncan Pritchard, *Epistemology*, Palgrave, 2016. For a
shorter introduction to the philosophy of knowledge, see

Paul Pardi, 'What is knowledge?', *Philosophy News*, 22 September 2011, https://www.philosophynews.com/post/2011/09/22/What-is-Knowledge.aspx.

3 John Hardwig, 'Epistemic dependence', *Journal of Philosophy*, 82, 1985, pp. 335–49.

4 Alvin Goldman, 'Experts: which one should you trust?', *Philosophy and Phenomenological Research*, 63.1, 2001, pp. 85–110.

5 John Stuart Mill, 'On liberty', in *On Liberty and Other Writings*, ed. Stefan Collini, Cambridge University Press, 1989, p. 53.

6 On Thomas Kuhn and COVID-19, see John Horgan, 'The coronavirus and right-wing postmodernism', *Scientific American*, 9 March 2020, https://blogs.scientificamerican.com/cross-check/the-coronavirus-and-right-wing-postmodernism/.

7 On Andrew Wakefield, see T. S. Sathyanarayana Rao and Chittaranjan Andrade, 'The MMR vaccine and autism: sensation, refutation, retraction, and fraud', *Indian Journal of Psychiatry*, 53.2, 2011, pp. 95–6.

8 On Wakefield and Trump, see Andrew Buncombe, 'Andrew Wakefield: how a disgraced UK doctor has remade himself in anti-vaxxer Trump's America', *The Independent*, 4 May 2018, https://www.independent.co.uk/news/world/americas/andrew-wakefield-anti-vaxxer-trump-us-mmr-autism-link-lancet-fake-a8331826.html.

9 On the lack of consensus among experts on COVID-19, see Neil Levy, Eric Schliesser and Eric Winsberg, 'Coronavirus: why it's dangerous to blindly "follow the science" when there's no consensus yet', *The Conversation*, 18 June 2020, https://theconversation.com/coronavirus-why-its-dangerous-to-blindly-follow-the-science-when-theres-no-consensus-yet-140980.

10 On social distancing and disagreements among experts, see Lena Ciric, 'One metre or two? The science behind social distancing', *The Conversation*, 18 June 2020, https://theconversation.com/one-metre-or-two-the-science-behind-social-distancing-139929.

11 On Francis Bacon's 'knowledge is power', see J. M. Rodriguez

García, '*Scientia potestas est* – knowledge is power: Francis Bacon to Michel Foucault', *Neohelicon*, 28, 2001, pp. 109–21, https://doi.org/10.1023/A:1011901104984.

12 On Michael Gove's famous claim that 'people in this country have had enough of experts', see https://www.ft.com/content/3be49734-29cb-11e6-83e4-abc22d5d108c.

13 On mathematical modelling and coronavirus, see https://bmcpublichealth.biomedcentral.com/articles/10.1186/s12889-020-08671-z.

14 On Sweden's controversial decision not to impose a strict lockdown in response to the COVID-19 pandemic, and the apology by Swedish state epidemiologist Anders Tegnell, see https://www.bbc.com/news/world-europe-52903717.

15 Maria Baghramian, quoted in Sylvia Thompson, 'Scientific advisers strive to be "honest brokers" in times of crisis', *The Irish Times*, 19 March 2020, https://www.irishtimes.com/news/science/scientific-advisers-strive-to-be-honest-brokers-in-times-of-crisis-1.4197587.

16 Maria Baghramian and Shane Bergin, 'Recreating climate of trust in experts essential for beating COVID-19', *The Irish Times*, 4 November 2020, https://www.irishtimes.com/opinion/recreating-climate-of-trust-in-experts-essential-for-beating-covid-19-1.4398927.

17 On trust in science and experts during the coronavirus crisis, see https://www.researchprofessionalnews.com/rr-news-europe-politics-2020-6-trust-in-the-time-of-coronavirus/.

18 Cicero, *De Officiis* 1.7.20.

19 On the raves in Manchester, see Josh Halliday, 'Six thousand people attend two illegal raves in Greater Manchester', *The Guardian*, 14 June 2020, https://www.theguardian.com/uk-news/2020/jun/14/six-thousand-people-attend-two-illegal-raves-greater-manchester.

20 On Onora O'Neill's views on trust and experts, see her interview at https://allea.org/interview-with-baroness-oneill-of-bengarve-we-see-a-great-deal-of-mud-thrown-at-most-forms-of-expertise-in-the-public-discourse-all-the-time/.

21 Joseph Raz, Tang Prize Text, 21 May 2020, https://www.tang-prize.org/en/media_detail.php?id=1382.

Notes

NOTES TO CHAPTER 8

1 Francesca Melandri, 'A letter to the UK from Italy: this is what we know about your future', *The Guardian*, 27 March 2020, https://www.theguardian.com/world/2020/mar/27/a-letter-to-the-uk-from-italy-this-is-what-we-know-about-yo ur-future.

2 On the rise of domestic abuse worldwide during the corona-virus lockdown, see Amanda Taub, 'A new Covid-19 crisis: domestic abuse rises worldwide', *New York Times*, 6 April 2020, https://www.nytimes.com/2020/04/06/world/corona virus-domestic-violence.html. See also https://www.cfr.org/ in-brief/double-pandemic-domestic-violence-age-covid-19. On the UN and the rise in domestic violence, see https:// news.un.org/en/story/2020/04/1061052.

3 On domestic violence in Ireland during the coronavirus lockdown, see Conor Lally, 'Domestic violence reports up 30% in some areas since lockdown, says Garda', *The Irish Times*, 27 April 2020, https://www.irishtimes.com/news/ crime-and-law/domestic-violence-reports-up-30-in-some -areas-since-lockdown-says-garda-1.4238362. For more recent statistics on domestic violence in Ireland in 2020, see Shauna Bowers, 'Calls to gardaí for domestic abuse and violence up 18% this year', *The Irish Times*, 28 October 2020, https://www.irishtimes.com/news/crime-and-law/ calls-to-garda%C3%AD-for-domestic-abuse-and-violence-u p-18-this-year-1.4393105.

4 On domestic violence in the UK during the coronavirus lock-down, see Mark Townsend, 'Revealed: surge in domestic vio-lence during Covid-19 crisis', *The Guardian*, 12 April 2020, https://www.theguardian.com/society/2020/apr/12/domest ic-violence-surges-seven-hundred-per-cent-uk-coronavirus.

5 Sally Rooney, *Normal People*, Faber and Faber, 2018. On the television adaptation of *Normal People* by the BBC, see https://www.bbc.com/news/entertainment-arts-52456148.

6 Susan Brison, *Aftermath: Violence and the Remaking of a Self*, Princeton University Press, 2002.

7 In Louise O'Neill's novel *Asking For It* (Riverrun, 2016), Emma is the survivor of a devastating sexual assault: 'I am

not falling apart. I am being ripped at the seams, my insides torn out until I am hollow.'

8 Brison, *Aftermath*, p. 40.

9 On the idea of violence as the violation of integrity, see Vittorio Bufacchi, *Violence and Social Justice*, Palgrave, 2007.

10 For a phenomenological analysis of violence, see Michael Staudigl, 'Towards a phenomenological theory of violence: reflections following Merleau-Ponty and Schutz', *Human Studies*, 30, 2007, pp. 233–53. On the idea that a phenomenological model makes it possible to see rape not as a property crime, but rather as an experienced attack on the very conditions of being a self and a subject in the world, see Louise du Toit, *A Philosophical Investigation of Rape: The Making and Unmaking of the Feminine Self*, Routledge, 2009.

11 On the long-term impact of violence, and how this changes the way we understand and define violence, see Vittorio Bufacchi and Jools Gilson, 'The ripples of violence', *Feminist Review*, 112, 2016, pp. 27–40.

Notes to Chapter 9

1 Michael D. Higgins quoted in *The Irish Times*, 8 July 2020, https://www.irishtimes.com/news/social-affairs/pandemic-has-shown-how-undervalued-frontline-workers-were-higgins-1.4299343.

2 On excess mortality in the UK, see Robert Booth, 'Excess deaths in UK under coronavirus lockdown pass 63,000', *The Guardian*, 9 June 2020, https://www.theguardian.com/society/2020/jun/09/excess-deaths-in-uk-under-coronavirus-lockdown-pass-63000. For international comparisons, see https://www.health.org.uk/news-and-comment/charts-and-infographics/understanding-excess-mortality-international-comparisons. See also https://ourworldindata.org/coronavirus/country/united-kingdom?country=~GBR.

3 On Ireland's excess mortality, see Rachel Lavin and Susan Mitchell, 'Ireland's COVID-19 excess deaths higher than EU norm', *Business Post*, 14 June 2020, https://www.business

post.ie/health/irelands-COVID-19-excess-deaths-higher-tha
n-eu-norm-7995a4be.

4 On New Zealand and coronavirus, see Sophie Cousins,
'New Zealand eliminates COVID-19', *The Lancet*, 9 May
2020, https://www.thelancet.com/journals/lancet/article/
PIIS0140-6736(20)31097-7/fulltext.

5 Philip Ball, 'Ten lessons of the COVID-19 pandemic', *New
Statesman*, 21 October 2020, https://www.newstatesman.
com/international/coronavirus/2020/10/ten-lessons-covid-
19-pandemic.

6 On why young people don't vote, see https://www.econo
mist.com/the-economist-explains/2014/10/29/why-young-
people-dont-vote.

7 Zygmunt Bauman, *Modernity and the Holocaust*, Polity,
1989.

8 For an overview of Brian Barry's political theory, see Vittorio
Bufacchi, 'Why political philosophy matters: reading Brian
Barry on social justice', *European Journal of Political
Theory*, 7.2, 2008, pp. 255–64.

9 Brian Barry and Marcel Wissenburg, 'The concept of the
state in political philosophy', *European Political Science*,
10, 2011, pp. 92–102.

10 On state authority leaking away to sub- and supranational
institutions, see also Marcel Wissenburg, *Political Pluralism
and the State*, Routledge, 2007.

11 Barry and Wissenburg, 'The concept of the state in political
philosophy', p. 97.

12 Chiara Cordelli, *The Privatized State*, Princeton University
Press, 2020.

13 On the problems and evils of neoliberalism, see Stephen
Metcalf, 'Neoliberalism: the idea that swallowed the
world', *The Guardian*, 18 August 2017, https://www.
theguardian.com/news/2017/aug/18/neoliberalism-the-idea-
that-changed-the-world.

14 Onora O'Neill, 'Do we really want things to go back to
normal post-COVID-19?', *The Irish Times*, 12 May 2020,
https://www.irishtimes.com/opinion/do-we-really-want-th
ings-to-go-back-to-normal-post-covid-19-1.4250554.

15 On Marx's theory of the state, see Rafael Khachaturian,

Notes

'The state', *Legal Form – A Forum for Marxist Analysis of Law*, 29 June 2020, https://legalform.blog/2020/06/29/the-state-rafael-khachaturian/.

16 Plato, *The Republic*, Book I, 343-D, Cosimo Classics, 2008, p. 18.

17 For a more in-depth analysis of the philosophy of taxation, see Martin O'Neill and Shepley Orr (eds), *Taxation: Philosophical Perspectives*, Oxford University Press, 2018.

18 Samuel Scheffler, 'Is economic inequality really a problem?', *New York Times*, 1 July 2020, https://www.nytimes.com/2020/07/01/opinion/economic-inequality-moral-philosophy.html. On the dangers and immorality of extreme inequality, see also Thomas Scanlon, *Why Does Inequality Matter?*, Oxford University Press, 2018.

19 On the limits of the market, see Debra Satz, *Why Some Things Should Not Be for Sale: The Limits of Markets*, Oxford University Press, 2010.

20 On Martin O'Neill's view that we need more radical reforms than changes to the tax system, see https://bostonreview.net/forum/taxing-superrich/martin-o%E2%80%99neill-economic-justice-requires-more-wealth-tax.

21 On basic income in Spain during COVID-19, see Guy Hedgecoe, 'Coronavirus: Spain experiments with basic income for most in need', *The Irish Times*, 28 May 2020, https://www.irishtimes.com/news/world/europe/coronavirus-spain-experiments-with-basic-income-for-most-in-need-1.4264895.

22 On basic income, see Philippe Van Parjis, *Real Freedom for All*, Oxford University Press, 1995; Philippe Van Parjis and Yannick Vanderborght, *Basic Income: A Radical Proposal for a Free Society and a Sane Economy*, Harvard University Press, 2017.

23 Jamie Cooke, Jurgen De Wispelaere and Ian Orton, 'COVID-19 and basic income', *Policy Network*, 12 October 2020, https://policynetwork.org/opinions/blogs/covid-19-and-basic-income/.

24 On predistribution, see Martin O'Neill, 'Predistribution: an unsnappy name for an inspiring idea', *The Guardian*, 12 September 2012, https://www.theguardian.com/commen

tisfree/2012/sep/12/ed-miliband-predistribution. See also Martin O'Neill, 'Power, predistribution, and social justice', *Philosophy*, 95.1, 2020, pp. 63–91.

25 On community wealth building, see Joe Guinan and Martin O'Neill, *The Case for Community Wealth Building*, Polity, 2020. See also their article 'Only bold state intervention will save us from a future owned by corporate giants', *The Guardian*, 6 July 2020, https://www.theguard ian.com/commentisfree/2020/jul/06/state-intervention-am azon-recovery-covid-19.

26 On the impact of coronavirus on Latin America, see Michael Stott and Andres Schipani, 'Poverty and populism put Latin America at the centre of pandemic', *Financial Times*, 14 June 2020, https://www.ft.com/content/aa84 f572-f7af-41a8-be41-e835bddbed5b.

NOTES TO EPILOGUE

1 On Hegel and the owl of Minerva, see Gary K. Browning, *Hegel and the History of Political Philosophy*, Palgrave, 1999. See also Lea Ypi, 'The owl of Minerva only flies at dusk, but to where? A reply to critics', *Ethics & Global Politics*, 6.2, 2013, pp. 117–34.

2 Martha Nussbaum, 'Public philosophy and international feminism', *Ethics*, 108.4, 1998, pp. 762–96.

3 On the philosophy of praxis, see Pete Thomas, 'Gramsci's Marxism: the "philosophy of praxis"', in M. McNally (ed.), *Antonio Gramsci*, Palgrave, 2005, pp. 97–117.

4 Bertrand Russell, *A History of Western Philosophy*, Simon and Schuster, 1945.

5 Sarah Caddy, Anne Moore, Connor Bamford, David Hunter, Derek Gatherer, Robert West and Susan Michie, 'A million deaths from coronavirus: seven experts consider key questions', *The Conversation UK*, 27 September 2020, https:// theconversation.com/a-million-deaths-from-coronavirus-se ven-experts-consider-key-questions-146085.

6 Joe Humphreys, 'Five lessons of Stoicism: what I learned from living for a week as a Stoic', *The Irish Times*, 29 October 2020, https://www.irishtimes.com/culture/five-

lessons-of-stoicism-what-i-learned-from-living-for-a-week-as-a-stoic-1.4392422. See also 'The Irish Times view on Stoicism in a pandemic: lessons on living', *The Irish Times*, 30 October 2020, https://www.irishtimes.com/opinion/edi torial/the-irish-times-view-on-stoicism-in-a-pandemic-less ons-on-living-1.4395523.

7 On John Locke, see *Two Treatises of Government*, ed. P. Laslett, Cambridge University Press, 1988.

8 On Thomas Jefferson and the Declaration of Independence, see https://web.archive.org/web/20140330160602/http:// www.ushistory.org/declaration/document/rough.htm.

9 On contemporary right-wing libertarianism, see Robert Nozick, *Anarchy, State and Utopia*, Blackwell, 1974. In recent years a left-wing interpretation of libertarianism has emerged; see Michael Otsuka, *Libertarianism Without Inequality*, Oxford University Press, 2005.

10 For a philosophical overview on the concept of rights, see https://plato.stanford.edu/entries/rights/.

11 On the idea that there can be obligations without rights, see Onora O'Neill, *Towards Justice and Virtue*, Cambridge University Press, 1996. See also her 'The dark side of human rights', *International Affairs*, 81.2, 2005, pp. 427–39.

12 On *primum non nocere*, and the more general obligation of non-maleficence, see Vittorio Bufacchi, 'Justice as non-maleficence', *Theoria*, 67.162, 2020, pp. 1–27.

Index

Index

Index

Index

Index